TOP
FITNESS
A D V I C E

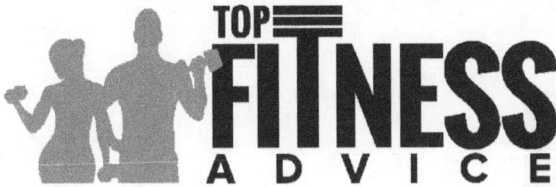

YOGA FOR WOMEN

14-Day Beginner's Guide to Yoga for Weight Loss, Stress Relief & Living Longer! (BONUS: 100 Yoga Poses with Instructions)

Amy Jenkins

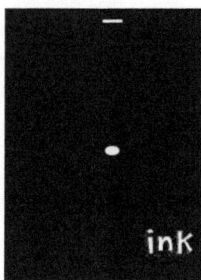

First published in 2017 by Venture Ink Publishing

For more information about the contents of this book or questions to the author, please contact Amy Jenkins at amy@topfitnessadvice.com

Disclaimer

This book provides wellness management information in an informative and educational manner only, with information that is general in nature and that is not specific to you, the reader. The contents of this book are intended to assist you and other readers in your personal wellness efforts. Consult your physician regarding the applicability of any information provided in this book to you.

Nothing in this book should be construed as personal advice or diagnosis, and must not be used in this manner. The information provided about conditions is general in nature. This information does not cover all possible uses, actions, precautions, side-effects, or interactions of medicines, or medical procedures. The information in this book should not be considered as complete and does not cover all diseases, ailments, physical conditions, or their treatment.

You should consult with your physician before beginning any exercise, weight loss, or health care program. This book should not be used in place of a call or visit to a competent health-care professional. You should consult a health care professional before adopting any of the suggestions in this book or before drawing inferences from it.

Any decision regarding treatment and medication for your condition should be made with the advice and consultation of a qualified health care professional. If you have, or suspect you have, a health-care problem, then you should immediately contact a qualified health care professional for treatment.

No Warranties: The author and publisher don't guarantee or warrant the quality, accuracy, completeness, timeliness, appropriateness or suitability of the information in this book, or of any product or services referenced in this book.

The information in this book is provided on an "as is" basis and the author and publisher make no representations or warranties of any kind with respect to this information. This book may contain inaccuracies, typographical errors, or other errors.

Table of Contents

Would you prefer to listen to my book, rather than read it?

Download the audiobook version for free!

If you go to the special link below and sign up to Audible as a new customer, you can get the audiobook version of my book completely free.

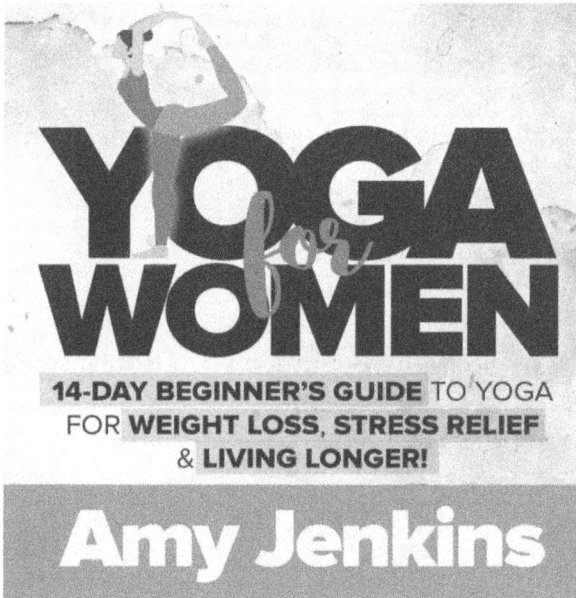

Go here to get your audiobook version for free:

TopFitnessAdvice.com/go/YogaWomen

Who is this book for?

Are you looking for a simple and safe solution, without drugs or harsh dieting, for weight loss, stress relief, and for a happier, even longer life?

Have you tried to start a yoga routine to help you lose those stubborn pounds, relax, and improve your overall health, only to find that your routine was ineffective, if not downright painful?

If so, this book is for you! We'll guide you through the simple steps you need to follow to start a yoga routine and make it successful and safe, and to ensure you know how to use yoga to lose weight and relieve your overall stress.

It doesn't matter your current physical condition, as the information we'll provide works for anyone in any shape, and whether or not you've ever tried yoga before.

What will this book teach you?

Yoga is probably one of the healthiest practices you can follow; it helps to stretch muscles you might otherwise overlook with basic workout routines, and also helps you to focus your mind while working out the body.

Yoga can help muscles bring in more blood and oxygen, so they can better support your exercise routines, helping you lose weight and keep it off.

Focusing your mind while performing your yoga routine also means relaxing and building concentration. This is why yoga is such a great stress reliever!

With flexible muscles, better blood circulation, and less tension, you may even find that your yoga routine makes your healthier overall and helps you live longer!

However, you won't enjoy any of these benefits if you don't know the basics of yoga, including the best poses for beginners and how to transition between poses.

You also need to know how to avoid making your yoga routine downright dangerous by stretching incorrectly, holding a pose too long, and other such common, beginner mistakes.

There are also a few simple tips and tricks you'll want to remember during your routine to make it even more effective and enjoyable!

This book will teach you everything you need to know about how to start a yoga routine as well as how to make it the best part of your day, and more effective for your own personal fitness goals.

Whether you've tried yoga before or are brand new to the practice, you're sure to learn everything you need to know to use yoga for weight loss, stress relief, better overall health, and even for a longer life!

Introduction

Understanding the Practice of Yoga Itself

So, just what is yoga? This is actually a very important question to consider, as many people are confused by the practice of yoga itself.

Some assume that yoga involves meditation or chanting, or that it's some type of spiritual practice. Some also may think that true yoga involves getting into very difficult positions and poses and holding them for a long time.

All of these assumptions are both true and false!

Let's talk first about yoga and meditation.

Yoga itself, on its own, doesn't involve meditation, but many practitioners find that it's helpful to set aside time to meditate after a yoga routine, and to involve a type of chant or mantra during this time. Going through a yoga routine will strengthen the muscles and make them more flexible, so you can easily sit still during meditation without muscle cramps or fatigue.

Concentrating or focusing during your yoga routine can also prepare you mentally for the focus you need to meditate once your routine is over.

However, note that these two practices are technically separate, so if you're not comfortable with the idea of meditation for any reason, you don't need to commit to this in order to enjoy the benefits of yoga.

Note, too, that chants and mantras used during yoga or meditation are not simply about making noise, but they allow the mind to focus on the sound you're making or the words you're repeating.

This is a way to enhance concentration and shut out outside distractions. Not many yoga practitioners use a chant or mantra, but it can help you to focus during certain poses.

Yoga is also not necessarily spiritual, although some parts of its practice may be used by certain religions and its adherents as a way to meditate, or to create a good physical response that is needed for prayer routines.

You can certainly use yoga in this way, choosing poses you need for strengthen the back and knees to support you in a prayer position, or to train you to block out distractions and focus on your own thoughts, as is needed for prayer. However, this too is not a requirement for benefiting from a yoga routine itself.

Also, the positions you get into and how long you hold them is up to you and each individual practitioner.

Some people will work their way up to a very difficult or challenging routine that may seem impossible to beginners, whereas you can get quite a bit of benefit from even the most basic of routines that involve simple poses that you hold for only a few seconds.

As your muscles flex and become more pliable and stronger, you may find that those seemingly odd and difficult poses are no longer difficult for you, and you may also realize the benefit of poses like headstands, standing on one foot, and the like.

In short, yoga is like many other routines you follow for physical fitness; it should work to benefit you and your goals, and should be a good match for your current fitness levels.

No matter how the practice began or how other people use it, yoga can have tremendous benefit for you when it comes to weight loss, flexibility, better blood circulation, better posture, relaxation, and improved overall health.

If you decide to add meditation or a spirituality to your yoga routine, this is certainly your decision, but don't assume that yoga itself is spiritual or that it should interfere with other religious beliefs and practices.

Discover Scientifically-Proven "Shortcuts" & "Hacks" to Lose Weight FASTER (With Very Little Effort)

For this month only, you can get Linda Westwood's best-selling & most popular book absolutely free – *Weight Loss Secrets You NEED to Know*.

Get Your FREE Copy Here:
TopFitnessAdvice.com/Extras

Discover scientifically-proven tips to help you lose weight faster and easier than ever before. With this book, readers were able to improve their weight loss results and fitness levels. So, it's highly recommended that you get this book, especially while it's free!

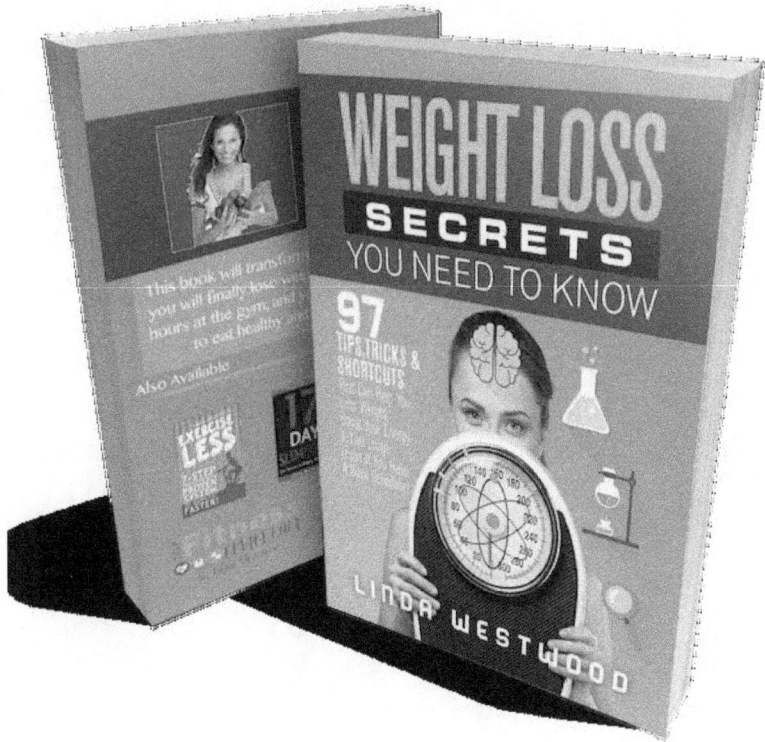

Get Your FREE Copy Here:

TopFitnessAdvice.com/Extras

Chapter 1

Yoga and Detoxifying

When you think of yoga, you may assume that your muscles are the only parts of your body that benefit.

In truth, yoga has many other benefits that you may not realize, including detoxifying your internal organs and major systems of the body. This can lead to better overall health and a longer life.

How does yoga help detoxify your body?

As you twist and stretch through different poses and positions, this can help to open up the organs such as the liver and lungs, and these work as natural filters for the body.

Twisting and stretching can then allow them to release more built-up toxins in your system, and function more optimally to filter out toxins.

Flexing and elongating your muscles can also mean that you have better posture and that your muscles are stretched properly, even when you're not following your routine.

If you are standing up properly and have good posture through the day, your stomach, intestines, and other such parts of your digestive system will receive more blood and oxygen and be able to eliminate waste more easily.

Note that your digestive system, including your belly, can hold the most amount of toxins and bacteria in your body.

When the muscles and organs that make up your digestive system do not have enough room internally for healthy blood flow, or when you are hunched over your belly because of poor posture, this bacteria can build up in your system.

By practicing yoga, you are stretching all parts of your body so that they function optimally and can better eliminate bacteria and other such harmful agents.

This stretching and flexing of muscles also allows for better blood flow through them, and through your entire circulatory system.

Blood brings needed vitamins, trace minerals, amino acids, and other such nutrients that are used to help the body repair and restore itself.

However, blood also works as something of a trash collector for the body, taking away dead cells and other such impurities. The more you stretch and increase that blood circulation, the more harmful agents will be removed from the body through your circulatory system.

Toxins won't build up around the liver and lungs, and your internal organs will get more of the nutrients needed to repair themselves and work more effectively.

Chapter 2

Yoga and Sleep

Let's take a look at the connection between yoga and sleep, and how this connection can mean less stress and even a longer, healthier life.

Sleep and Stress

One of the most important parts of alleviating stress and tension is getting a good night's sleep.

Sleep allows your body's systems to repair and restore themselves, since they slow down while you sleep.

You are still digesting food, breathing in and out, and everything else you do during the day, but this slowdown means less use of your internal organs and muscles. In turn, your body can then concentrate on repairing your systems.

This repairing and restoring usually happens during your deepest sleep, so staying up late, tossing and turning so that you only get "light" sleep, or waking up often during the night can interfere with this process.

This can actually happen without you even being aware of it; muscle aches or poor blood circulation may mean waking up just long enough to shift positions, and then you fall asleep again.

However, this is enough interruption of sleep to also interfere with your body's process of restoration.

When you do get a good night's sleep, you feel healthier when you awaken as your muscles and internal organs have been repaired and strengthened.

In turn, you may have more energy, and your body has metabolized all those stress hormones and chemicals in your system.

Getting a good night's sleep can also help you to think more clearly throughout the day. Remember that the brain is an organ like all the others in your body, so it also needs to be repaired and restored in order to function properly.

The cells of the brain actually get repaired during sleep, so you can concentrate better during the day. Your brain may also work more effectively, so you have better problem-solving skills and clearer thinking overall.

If one of your causes of stress is struggling to keep up with the demands of your job or just juggling many responsibilities at once, having a healthier brain that functions better may actually help alleviate this stress!

A lack of good sleep can add to your stress as you may experience daytime drowsiness, mood swings, anger, and many other negative emotions, usually brought on by those stress hormones that your body has not metabolized at night.

Your brain may also be struggling to function so that you lack concentration and problem-solving abilities, and this also adds to stress; you forget simple things, cannot accomplish things as you should, and find it difficult to keep up with the demands of your job and family.

Simply being tired itself can also make you feel stressed and anxious!

Shutting Out Thoughts While Doing Yoga

Many people who start a yoga routine report that they enjoy better sleep; they can fall asleep quickly and stay asleep all night.

This is due to a few factors; one is the relaxation you may enjoy with yoga, as you focus on your body and your movements and shut off outside distractions.

Your mind has this peaceful, calm break during the day so that it can begin to relax and rest and be ready for sleep at night.

Learning how to shut out these distractions during the day can also help you to do the same at night, when it's time for bed.

If you're the type who tosses and turns, struggling to get to sleep because your mind is racing or suddenly feels overwhelmed with problems, learning how to focus on your feelings and relax your mind can help you fall asleep as soon as your head hits the pillow.

You may also be less likely to wake up in the middle of the night from tense and stressful thoughts that go through your head while you sleep.

Yoga and the Muscles

Another factor when it comes to yoga and better sleep is that stretching the muscles allows them to relax, so your whole body is relaxed. In turn, you're not as tense and sore at night.

Many people have a hard time falling asleep because they have pain in the lower back or shoulders, or have leg cramps.

This pain may be relatively minor so that it's not as noticeable throughout the day, but once you're trying to get to sleep at night, you suddenly feel stiff and uncomfortable and cannot seem to settle down and get to sleep.

When you stretch your muscles during a yoga routine, that added blood flow and extra oxygen you take in, as well as the toxins that are collected from this blood circulation, makes your muscles feel healthier and less tense.

If you notice that your back seems to tense up or your shoulders and neck just cannot relax when you put head to pillow at night, a basic yoga routine can alleviate this.

Stretching and flexing the muscles and making them stronger also means that they won't be as worn out from supporting your weight all day.

If you have poor posture, you could be putting too much weight on muscles that are not meant to support the body's weight so that those muscles are stiff and sore at night.

Muscles that aren't flexed and strong may also simply struggle to hold your body upright, so that you feel aches and pains when you finally get off your feet at night.

Those muscles may also want to stay cramped and wrapped up as they are during the day, and may not be comfortable in a reclining position. This may cause you to wake up during the night as you shift position, or as the muscles struggle to adjust to new positions.

By stretching and strengthening muscles with yoga, they won't be so worn from supporting you during the day and will be better able to relax at bedtime. This, too, will mean a better night's sleep and more rest overall.

I hope that you are enjoying this book so far, and if you could spare 30 seconds, I would greatly appreciate you leaving a review on Amazon.com.

Chapter 3

Yoga and Increased Blood Circulation

Stretching your muscles and getting into various poses and positions with yoga can help to improve your overall blood circulation.

When muscles are stretched, they are better able to let blood flow through them. When you improve your posture with yoga, you are also letting more blood flow through your veins and arteries and other parts of your circulatory system.

Standing on your head or just bending into various positions also encourages more blood flow to parts of the body that may not always get so much blood; headstands increase blood circulation to the brain, and bending forward allows for more blood in the upper back and shoulders as well as the neck.

There are many benefits to this increased blood flow you experience with yoga. Let's note a few of them here.

Feeding and nourishing cells

Blood picks up vital nutrients from the digestive system, including all the vitamins, minerals, amino acids, and other trace elements that are extracted from food as it's digested.

The blood then also picks up an oxygen molecule from the lungs, and delivers these to each cell of the body. These nutrients form the building blocks of new, healthy cells, and they help to repair any damage that is done from everyday activities.

They also repair damage done to bones, muscles, tendons, and all other parts of your body that is done by harmful elements from pollution, toxins in your system, and the like.

Without healthy blood flow, your muscles and organs will break down as you age but not be repaired as easily.

In turn, they simply won't work as well, so your brain may struggle to think and concentrate, your muscles may struggle to hold you upright, and your bones may become more and more brittle over time.

This is also one reason why yoga can actually help you to live longer. Remember that the heart, lungs, and other vital parts of the body are muscles and organs that break down as your age, eventually leading to your death.

The stronger you can keep your heart, your lungs, your digestive system, and other such important systems in the body, the stronger you will be over time. This can actually lead to a longer, healthier life!

Chapter 4

Yoga Benefits Your Bones

When you stretch to reach each pose in yoga, you are mostly working the muscles of the body, as well as the spine.

However, this also involves stretching aligning the bones properly. You may notice that, during a yoga routine, you don't simply twist into different poses or hold those poses, but your body curves and reaches for a new position in gentle, fluid forms.

This helps to keep those bones in proper alignment. They aren't bending at the joint or being twisted out of place, but are being stretched and flexed along with your muscles.

There are a few benefits to stretching your bones along with your muscles.

One is that you may find you have less risk of arthritis or other joint conditions, as you're keeping your joints flexible.

You're also learning to avoid putting undue stress on your joints when you follow a yoga routine; your posture can improve and you may find that you naturally stretch your leg muscles when standing, which then alleviates some pressure on your bones.

Stronger bones are also needed for a healthy workout routine for weight loss. Your bones absorb some of the impact of your steps and other activities, so if they're somewhat weak or out of alignment, this can allow your joints and muscles to absorb that impact.

In turn, you can be at greater risk for tearing a ligament or other such damage, or for feeling sore and stiff.

Persistent workouts can also result in painful stress fractures of the bones; avoiding this risk is another reason to follow a healthy yoga routine, especially if you're looking to exercise for weight loss as well.

Once again, thank you for reading this book, and I hope you're getting a lot of valuable information. I would greatly appreciate it if you could take 30 seconds to leave me a review for this book on Amazon.com.

Chapter 5

Yoga and Weight Loss

Yoga itself will burn some calories, as you're not spending your entire routine sitting down, motionless. However, yoga in of itself is not actually meant for serious weight loss, as the motions you go through during yoga are meant to be gentle and fluid.

This doesn't mean you don't lose weight when you start a yoga routine, and yoga can actually be a very important key to losing weight and keeping it off for good.

As a matter of fact, if you've tried every diet out there and every workout routine you could find but still haven't lost weight, or need to give up that routine before not too long simply because it's uncomfortable if not downright painful, yoga may be just what you've been missing.

Consider how yoga can be so important when it comes to losing weight and keeping it off for good.

Yoga Makes You Strong

One reason that yoga can help with weight loss is that stretching your muscles and skin, and keeping your bones in better alignment, can mean being strong enough to support a workout regimen.

Very often people stop a workout routine or stop exercising altogether because their body simply isn't strong enough to support that routine. They may experience some aches and pains or find that they get too tired even from simple walking or aerobic activity.

If this has happened to you, it may be that you're overexerting yourself and aren't yet strong enough to manage all that movement and bouncing around with an aerobic routine, and it may also be that you need to stretch your muscles and make them flexible.

Flexible muscles are getting in more blood and oxygen so they can repair themselves more readily after a workout, and they become stronger overall.

Being flexible also means less risk of pulling a muscle, twisting a joint, tearing a ligament, or suffering any other type of sports injury that can interfere with your weight loss plans. You are more able to bend and stretch and absorb the impact of each step when you work your muscles and make them strong and flexible with yoga.

Yoga and Energy

The healthier blood flow you enjoy after following a workout routine may also mean more energy, as you'll be feeding your body's cells the nourishing vitamins and trace minerals you need for energy. This can also help your blood to better absorb glucose or sugar, so that your blood sugar levels remain healthy.

Of course, if you have diabetes or any other blood sugar condition, and are taking medication of any sort, you always want to ensure your doctor is monitoring your health and never stop taking your medication without his or her direction.

However, if you often put off a workout simply because you're tired and fatigued or don't have the energy to even start, a simple and basic yoga routine can be the solution.

You'll get the blood flowing and get your muscles working and feel more energy throughout the day, and for when it's time to jump into your aerobics class or go out for a jog.

Since yoga can also help you to sleep at night, as we've already discussed, this may also help you to have the energy needed for a good workout.

Rather than feeling groggy throughout the day and too fatigued to hit the gym after working, or feeling that mid-afternoon slump right when you were planning heading out to the gym, you'll feel rested and energized and will have the energy needed to work out and finally lose weight.

Enjoying this book?

Check out our other best sellers!

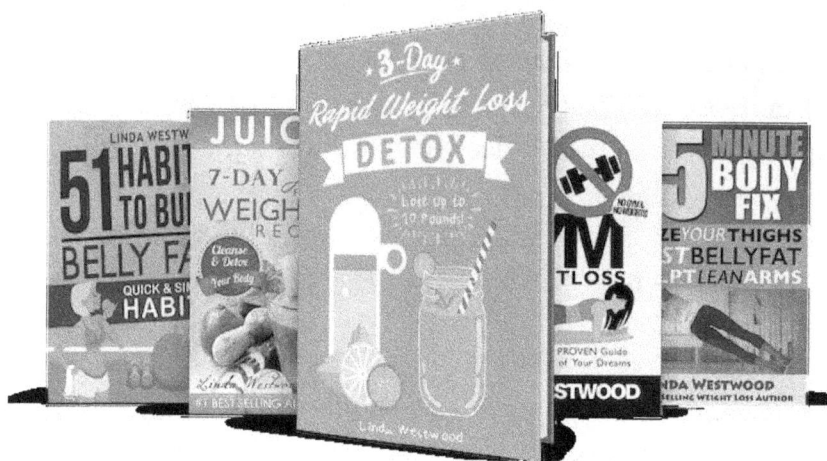

Get your next book on sale here:

TopFitnessAdvice.com/go/books

Chapter 6

Combining Yoga, Aerobics, and Pilates

You may see that yoga is often combined with other routines, such as aerobics or Pilates, and wonder if these routines are beneficial and safe, and as good as standard yoga itself.

There is no right or wrong answer to this; your workout routine needs to be effective for your goals, whether that's weight loss, increased flexibility, stamina, or developing muscles.

Telling you what you should or should not do with your basic yoga routine and poses is like saying you should or should not have eggs for dinner versus a steak!

There are pros and cons to combining yoga poses and moves with other workout routines; for example, going from a deep, static stretch to a quick movement can mean burning lots of calories, as your body needs to work harder to support this type of interval training.

Using yoga poses with a Pilates routine can mean stretching your muscles and then also building muscle tone, as Pilates uses your body's own weight for resistance training. Your muscles can then get a great workout while still safely stretching and enjoying the benefits of added blood and oxygen flow.

As with any workout routine, you need to ensure that you're being safe about your movements; you never want to overextend your muscles, use a jerking motion when twisting, or bounce so severely that you put undue stress on your joints or back.

If you do want to combine your yoga moves with another routine, it might be good to follow a routine created by an expert, either online or with a DVD, so you know you'll be safe and your workout will be effective.

Others who are considering purchasing this book would love to know what you think. If you could spare a few seconds, they would greatly appreciate reading an honest review from you. Simply visit the page on Amazon.com.

Chapter 7

Yoga and Your Attitude

How is it that yoga changes or affects your attitude? There are a few things to consider about a yoga routine and your way of thinking, especially when it comes to thinking about your health, both physical and emotional.

One Small Step

Very often people want to make changes that will benefit their overall health and wellbeing, but don't know where and how to start. They may also be very overwhelmed, thinking of how they'll need to make changes to their diet, work out, reduce stress, go to bed earlier and so on. Being overwhelmed can mean giving up on making any changes before you even begin!

Taking one small step toward better health can often be all that motivation you need to take another step, and then another. The key is to choose something manageable when starting out with making those changes, rather than trying to follow a new diet, workout regime, and daily schedule at once.

Yoga is certainly one small step that people can take to get them working toward many other goals; if you've come across this book because you're a beginner with yoga and know you also need to make some other, healthier changes in your life, then you can certainly understand that!

Yoga is easy enough for anyone to follow and use every single day, no matter your current fitness levels. Taking this one small

35

step of caring for your body by stretching and flexing muscles in a simple yoga routine can be just what you need to take the next step of joining a gym or trying some Pilates, or going for a long walk every day.

Forced Relaxation

The term forced relaxation may seem like a contradiction; how can something be relaxing if it's forced? This term refers to being forced to set aside time to focus your mind and calm your body.

In this instance, following a yoga routine doesn't mean something unpleasant, but it means having a specific time when you will relax, turn off the television, not let yourself be distracted by emails and the kids, and concentrate on your movements alone.

This type of forced relaxation can be what you need to eliminate and alleviate stress; too often, a person wants to shut out disquieting thoughts and relax their mind, but trying to do that without a set time and a distraction on which to focus can make it nearly impossible.

When you follow a yoga routine, you need to focus on your movements and your form, and note how long you're holding a pose, the next pose you'll move into, and so on. This can help your mind relax as you concentrate on improving your overall physical wellbeing while shutting out distracting and disquieting thoughts.

Chapter 8

Why So Many Beginner Yoga Routines Fail

If you've tried yoga before but found that you couldn't stick with it or that it seemed too challenging, and then gave up on following that routine, you're certainly not alone.

Let's note a few common reasons why beginner yoga routines fail so you can see if you've made any of these mistakes, and can avoid them with your new yoga routine!

Curving, Not Bending or Pounding

If you've tried yoga and found that your back or other joints and areas of the body were very painful afterwards, you may not be moving into each position or switching poses properly.

When you follow a yoga routine, your body should gently curve and flow into position and when you change a pose. You never want to bend your body; for example, if you try a pose that has you look upward and then stretch your hands behind your back, you want to have a curve in your back rather than bending at the waist.

Curving your body stretches muscles gently, whereas bending the back and other joints simply puts pressure and weight on those areas.

You also want to avoid pounding, bouncing, or otherwise putting sudden pressure on your joints.

A pose that involves a twist, such as twisting at the waist, should never include bouncing back and forth or a sudden, jarring movement into that position. This won't stretch the muscles any more effectively and can simply result in injury and resultant pain.

Trying Complicated, Advanced Poses

When you look at yoga poses online, you may assume that, to follow a real yoga routine, you need to get into very difficult positions. This might include a headstand, standing on one foot while leaning forward, and the like.

These types of positions can be very challenging for a beginner, so it's not unusual to get discouraged and think about giving up on your routine when you realize you cannot even get into such a position, much less hold it for several seconds!

While you want to challenge yourself with your yoga, following such a program is like any other fitness routine; start with what is manageable for you and slowly work your way to something more challenging.

Rather than giving up, simply note if you're making progress each week for how close you can get to certain poses or for how long you can hold them.

At the same time, remember that even the most basic, beginner poses and yoga routines will have tremendous benefits for your muscles, blood circulation, and overall health.

Trying to Rush Through

When you stretch your muscles, your body needs several seconds to get fresh blood and oxygen to those elongated spots.

If you rush through your yoga routine, you may improve your flexibility a slight bit and may have a small increase in your overall blood circulation, but may not see as many benefits as you would if you took your time and slowly moved through positions, and held them for several seconds.

If you tend to rush through your yoga routine because you don't have time in your schedule, consider going through a shorter list of poses and holding them for several seconds, rather than trying to reach a few dozen positions in one routine. This can keep your yoga workout effective no matter how much you have to devote to it.

I hope you have learned something from this book so far and would greatly appreciate it if you could leave an honest review on Amazon.com.

Chapter 9

Keeping Yoga Safe

One great advantage of yoga is that it involves little to no impact, when done properly. You gently transition from one pose to another, without slamming onto the ground as you do with aerobics or other workout routines.

However, this doesn't mean that yoga is always safe, as you need to ensure you remember some basics about the practice itself and keep yourself safe during your workout.

Be Careful of Slipping

A nice yoga mat can keep you from having to get onto an unhygienic floor when going through your routine, but note that most yoga mats can easily slip and slide on carpeting, stone, and tile.

The mat might also cause pressure on your knees, ankles, hips, or wrists as you try to stop this slippage. You could twist a joint or even tear ligament if you're not careful!

To avoid this slipping, be sure to wear shoes with good tread on the bottom that will grip the mat and keep it in place as you move from one position to another, or do your yoga barefoot.

Avoid wearing socks alone, as the smooth surface of the socks can actually make this slipping worse!

Also, perform your movements slowly so you can ensure you have proper balance and are keeping the mat in place from one position to another.

Proper Support

While yoga may stretch the spine and back, you don't want to put undue stress on these areas in particular.

For example, if you hold a pose on your back with your legs in the air or curved behind you, over your head, you always want to hold your hips and provide your spine with support as you curve out of this position.

Otherwise, you will be putting all your bodyweight on that curving spine and could cause damage to the discs of the back.

Remember this point also when you're doing handstands or any such movement with the head and neck. Hold yourself up by your hands, not your head, and never put undue pressure on the neck no matter the pose.

If a position seems uncomfortable or you feel pain in that area after your routine, give yourself more support or double-check that you're performing that movement properly.

Hydration and Eating

Be careful about eating big meals before a yoga routine; even a simple and basic routine will involve some stretching and bending of the core, or the stomach area. With a lot of food in your stomach, you may get acid reflux, or have your stomach acids regurgitate back up into your throat.

Having a lot of water in your stomach can also be very uncomfortable during a yoga routine, for the same reasons. You may feel pressure on the stomach and bladder, and may not be able to hold certain poses for very long.

However, it's good to ensure proper hydration after your yoga routine. Twisting and bending will release toxins from the body, as already discussed, and more water will help to flush these toxins from your system.

Water is also needed by your body for healthy blood circulation; since yoga will help your body to increase blood flow, you want to support this added circulation by having lots of water after your yoga routine.

Chapter 10

Your 14-Day Beginner's Yoga Routine

Now that you know everything there is to know about the benefits of yoga and how to use it for weight loss, and how to keep yourself safe during your routine, let's start out with a basic, 14-day beginner's yoga routine you can follow.

Be sure to reference the yoga poses included in this book so you know the terms used here and can follow these routines safely, and decide when you want to mix up these poses and create your own routine.

Day One, Two, and Three

Start with corpse pose, keeping yourself still on the mat, feeling your back and legs staying active but relaxed. Give yourself several seconds in this pose, to focus your mind and start breathing deeply.

Move into knees to chest pose. It may be difficult to hold your knees tightly against your chest the first few times you do this, but keep them as bent as possible and wrap your arms around your legs to keep them in position. Keep your hips on the floor so you aren't stretching your spine out of alignment.

Next, move into reclined goddess pose. Again, you may not be able to lower your legs and knees all the way to the mat, but hold them as wide as possible while keeping your feet on the ground, touching each other. Gently press down on your inner thighs to help this stretch. Keep your back active but relaxed.

With your feet together, push yourself up with your hands and then stretch forward into cobbler pose. Be sure your back is gently stretched and not simply bent at the waist; you want to flex the spine but not put pressure on your back in order to hold yourself up.

With your hands still on the mat, move your legs behind you to reach plank pose. Your back will be working hard to keep you in this pose, but don't let it collapse as this will put pressure on the back. Lower yourself to your knees for a few seconds if you don't have the strength to hold yourself upright with your arms alone.

Move your hands and feet to the corners of the mat and gently let your upper body curve downward so you come into downward dog.

If you can't flatten your feet on the mat, do the best you can to stretch your leg muscles. Let your upper body curve downward, without holding your shoulders and neck tense. Your back should feel stretched but not overextended.

Gently step your right foot forward as far as you can, then give yourself a moment to shift your weight and maintain your balance.

Step your left foot forward, again taking a moment to regain your balance, then bend forward and reach behind your ankles, wrapping your arm around your leg for standing forward bend.

Try to keep your upper body as close to your legs as possible for the most stretch.

Put your hands back up at the corners of the mat and put your feet back, returning to downward dog. Hold this position for several seconds again, continuing to stretch those leg muscles.

Keeping your hands and feet in place, gently bend your midsection forward and curve your upper body back, coming into cobra pose. Don't curve your upper body back too far so that it's uncomfortable, but be sure you are curving and not simply lifting your body off the ground.

You should feel your lower back folding or pushing down toward your abdomen. Lower yourself from this position by gently curving down, first your belly, then shoulders, then neck. Pause while on the mat, then curve yourself back into this position and hold it again.

From cobra pose, lower your knees to the mat and slide your hands back so that your body is in a square, your hands under your shoulders. Gently bend your back into cat pose. Be sure you keep your neck lowered so that the top of your head points downward, or else you'll be putting pressure on the neck.

Returning to your neutral or beginning position, keep your hands in place and then gently bend your knees so that you lean backwards, sitting on your heels. Keep your hands and arms outstretched in front of you so you come to child's pose.

If you can't bend your knees or legs all the way, just bend as far as you can to stretch those leg muscles. You should also feel a stretch in your back as you reach forward, and remember to keep your head tucked down, then reach your arms back so your hands are pointed behind you.

Putting your arms back in front of you, balance yourself with your hands as you straighten up and return to a downward dog pose.

Move from downward dog to another standing forward bend. Hold this for several seconds, and focus on whether or not this second time holding this pose is now easier. This will tell you that your routine is working!

Next, gently roll yourself up; don't simply straighten up, but roll the waist and then upper body, then the neck and head, so you're standing straight up, in mountain pose.

Hold this pose for several seconds as you concentrate on your back, feeling the muscles stretch and flex. Focus on your posture and note if you need to straighten up and alleviate pressure on the lower back and keep your head and neck in better alignment.

Gently move into half lotus tree; shift your weight to one foot and gain your balance, then lift the other foot and tuck it onto that opposite leg. Once you've gained your balance again, gently lift your arms into the air. If you fall out of this position, give yourself time to regain your balance and try again.

After switching legs and holding the pose, put your feet back on the ground and then step outward, into wide leg stance. Feel the inside of your thighs stretch. Be sure you mind your posture and keep yourself upright and balanced.

Step back so you're again in mountain pose and breathe deeply, concentrating on your posture and balance. Hold this pose and then you're done!

Day Four

Start in mountain pose, but standing on one edge of your yoga mat, with it stretched out before you. Take a few seconds to mind your posture and balance, feeling yourself stretched from head to toe.

Widen your stance so your feet are on the edges of the mat, then lean forward and put your palms on the mat, gently walking yourself forward to downward dog. Again, be sure you're hanging your head and not holding tension in your neck. Keep your back active but relaxed, not tense.

Gently curve your body downward into cobra pose and feel the back stretch. Hold this position for several seconds before curving your upper body down onto the mat, and then returning to cobra pose again.

Come out of cobra pose by bending your knees backward so you can then stand up, curling your back up until you're standing upright.

Shift your weight to your right leg, then bend at the waist, keeping your upper body straight so your body forms a ninety-degree angle while you reach onto the ground with your left hand, putting your left palm flat onto the mat. Extend your left leg straight behind you, so you come into half-moon pose.

Hold your right arm out so it helps with balance. Remember that your upper body should be in a ninety-degree angle throughout this pose, not curved. Let your back stretch but don't tense those muscles.

Bring your leg down and gently roll up and return to mountain pose, giving yourself another minute to stretch your back and feel your strength and posture.

Next, step forward gently with your right foot, keeping the left foot planted in place, and bend the right knee, leaning back on your right heel, as you reach up into high lunge pose. Feel your back stretch while your leg muscles support you, not your knees.

Return to mountain pose and breathe. Lower yourself onto the mat gently and cross your legs, coming into easy pose. Sit this way for several minutes, letting your back stretch while you feel your legs and knees flexing.

Uncross your legs and gently curve yourself up so that you're standing up again. Gently come into a standing back bend pose. Be sure you're curving your lower back inward, and not just bending your head back to look up at the ceiling. Gently curve yourself back into an upright position, and then repeat this pose.

After returning to an upright position, curve to one side for a standing side stretch. Mind your weight and balance as you do this; feel the stretch reach all the way down your legs and not just your back. Repeat this position for both sides.

Step your feet apart and put your hands on the mat again, returning to downward dog.

Next, step forward with your right foot, gain your balance, then step forward with your left foot, and reach behind your ankles for standing forward bend.

Gently curve out of this position for mountain pose, and hold it for several seconds as you tune into your leg and back muscles and breathe deeply.

Day Five and Six

For days five and six, repeat day the routine you followed on days one through three. This will give your body a chance to rest from the more challenging poses you just followed on the previous day, while still giving you a deep workout.

Day Seven

Day seven will work on your midsection more than anything, so be sure you haven't eaten for an hour or so before your routine and don't have too much water in your belly either.

Start with corpse pose to get yourself aligned and focused on your body. Keep your legs active but relaxed, your back also active and not simply collapsed into the mat. Move into a seated forward bend to stretch the legs even more.

Curve your back up to a seated position, the curve back into a one-legged staff pose. Return to a seated position and come into a seated angle bend, stretching for your toes as much as possible as you gently curve your upper body forward.

Tuck a leg inward for hand to knee pose, keeping the back gently curved. Straighten the legs and stand up to get into a runner's lunge with a twist.

Gently drop down into Zen pose and hold this for several minutes, then return to corpse pose for rest.

Day Eight, Nine, and Ten

Days eight through ten should repeat the routine you followed for the first three days, for more work on the legs and balance.

Day Eleven

Start in an easy Zen pose to mind your posture and balance, and to breathe deeply. Step out of this position and get into horse pose, working your inner thigh muscles.

Step into a runner's lunge with a twist, holding this for as long as you feel the leg muscles stretch. Be sure to switch sides and hold them both equally. Your legs should be easier to stretch and your balance should be better on day eleven.

Next, step back to the edge of your mat and lean forward, palms on the ground, walking yourself into downward dog position. Gently curve from this position to cobra pose. If you can manage it, pick your hands up for cobra II pose, and feel the lower back muscles stretch and contract to loosen up.

Curve back into downward dog and then step into standing forward bend. Curve your body back up into mountain pose and breathe deeply. End in reverse Namaste.

Day Twelve and Thirteen

Repeat your routine from the first three days for a general stretch and to concentrate on your leg muscles and the progress you're making in getting them flexed and pliable.

Day Fourteen

Day fourteen is a good chance to work in some advanced yoga moves and really challenge yourself, now that you're stretched and flexible! Start with corpse pose, then move into a boat pose to work the abdominals. Lean back for a reclined goddess pose and push the legs outward, really stretching them as far as possible.

Roll yourself up and squat into an awkward pose, holding those inner thigh muscles and keeping the back straight and active, but not tense. Then get down into a wide squat pose and hold this, pushing those leg muscles to their max.

Now try a crane position by leaning forward onto your hands and gently stepping your knees onto your triceps. If you can't hold your balance, keep your head on the mat while you work up to this pose.

Step back and then lie back onto the mat, rolling yourself backward into a plow pose. Feel your spine stretch as much as possible. Roll out of this position and put your hands back onto the mat, lifting yourself into a crab pose.

Lie back down into a reclined hero pose, feeling your belly and chest open up.

Roll over into a downward dog position to flex those leg muscles. Before ending your routine, choose one very challenging position you want to try, such as the eight angle pose or firefly pose.

Work this position into the end of this routine, then finish with a reverse Namaste to relax and rest the muscles, and you're done!

Don't forget to share your thoughts on this book by leaving a review on Amazon.com. It takes just a few seconds.

Conclusion

Hopefully this book has given you all the tools you need to follow a basic, beginner's yoga routine and to create your own routine by adding in those challenging poses at the end.

Remember to stay safe when doing yoga, to try something new and different each time you're on the mat, and to shut out all distractions so you can focus on your form.

If you do all that, you'll have a great yoga routine that will be easy enough to follow when starting out, and which will really help to build flexibility, help you to lose weight, help you to ease your stress, and even help you to live a long and happy life!

Discover Scientifically-Proven "Shortcuts" & "Hacks" to Lose Weight FASTER (With Very Little Effort)

For this month only, you can get Linda Westwood's best-selling & most popular book absolutely free – *Weight Loss Secrets You NEED to Know*.

Get Your FREE Copy Here:

TopFitnessAdvice.com/Extras

Discover scientifically-proven tips to help you lose weight faster and easier than ever before. With this book, readers were able to improve their weight loss results and fitness levels. So, it's highly recommended that you get this book, especially while it's free!

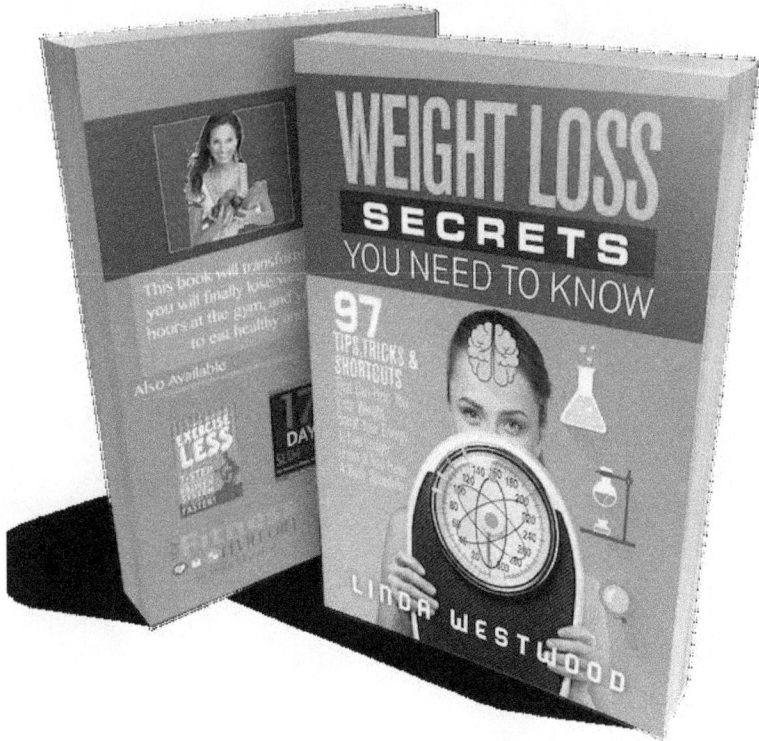

Get Your FREE Copy Here:

TopFitnessAdvice.com/Extras

100 Yoga Poses

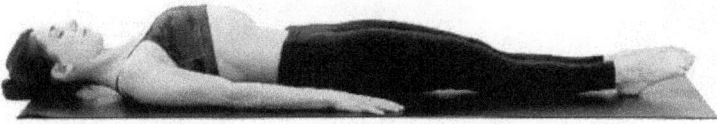

Corpse Position

This position may look very simple, but the purpose of starting or ending a routine with corpse position is to tune into your muscles and make sure they're stretched, and that your body is properly aligned. Note the model's toes; pointing them flexes the leg muscles and starts that stretch.

The back is also still active, though not rigid; don't simple collapse onto the mat in corpse position, but keep yourself firmly in place, noting all your muscles and your overall alignment. Focus on your breathing and your stomach and lungs moving in and out with each breath.

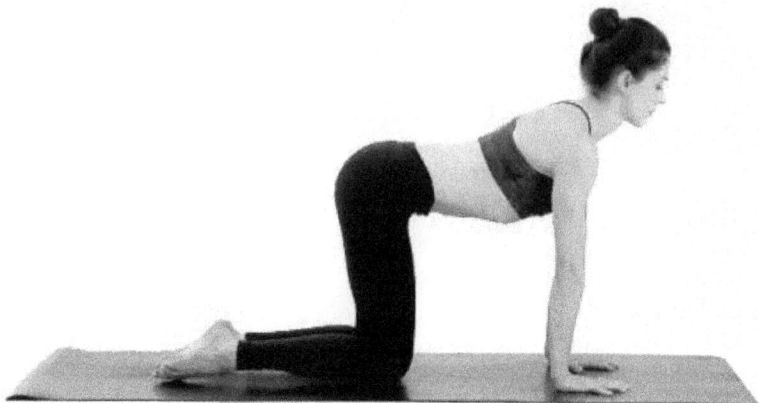

Table Top Pose

This pose helps to flex and relax the back muscles, undoing tensions and stress from poor posture or from staying in one position for too long throughout the day. Note the slight curve in the back, which helps to work those muscles and get the blood flowing.

In table top pose, be sure your leg muscles are firm and flexed; you don't want to support your body's weight on your knees, as this causes damage to the joints. Your hips and knees should also be in alignment, so avoid pushing backward and bending the knees.

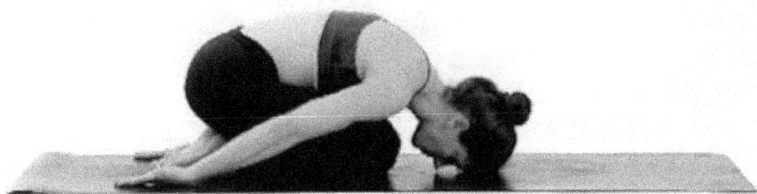

Child's Pose

This pose really stretches the muscles of the legs and back and helps to firm the buttocks as well. When starting with a yoga routine, you may not be able to fold your knees completely, so hold this pose only as deeply as you can manage until those muscles become more flexible.

Be sure you feel your back stretched but don't hold any tension in your neck; relax the neck and head as you rest your forehead on the mat, holding yourself in position with your leg muscles.

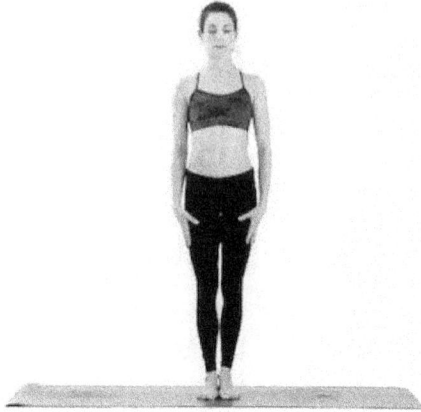

Mountain Pose

This pose may look very simple, but when standing up, you need to note the flexibility in your legs and back and concentrate on how your weight is balanced between your legs.

This pose allows you to feel any slumping or slouching in your posture, and easily stretch the back muscles by standing upright without being rigid. This also prepares the legs for more challenging poses.

Concentrate on your feet gripping the mat and the ground underneath you, so you can shift positions easily without swaying or falling off balance.

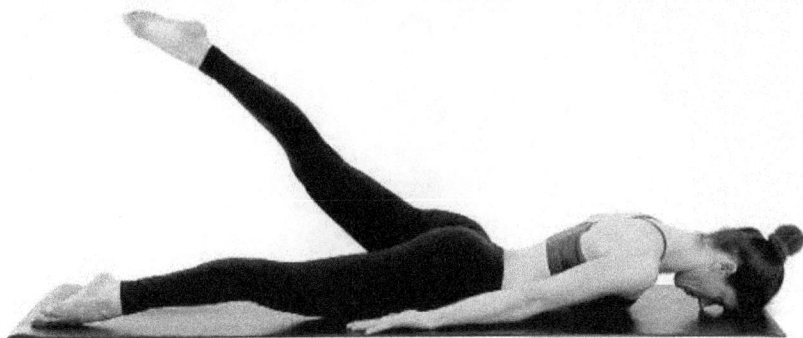

Half Locust Pose

This pose tenses the buttocks and helps build strong muscles in the backs of the legs, as well as inside the thighs and those hard-to-reach muscles that are often overlooked with other workout routines.

Keep your forehead to the mat so you don't pull on either side of the body, arms behind you and still active, not simply collapsing your upper body to the floor.

Be sure your lower back is active but not tensed or holding your body weight. All the exertion for this pose should be done with the legs and buttocks, not the back or neck.

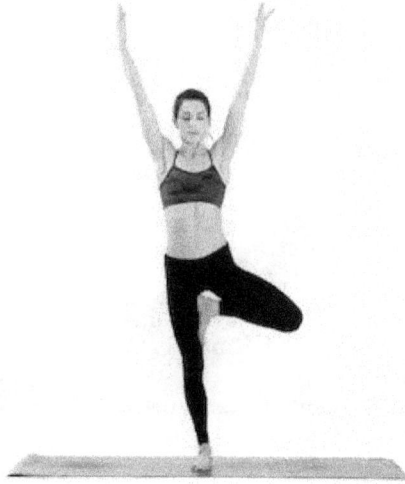

Half Lotus Tree

This pose not only stretches and flexes the leg muscles, but it also stretches the upper body and builds proper posture and balance.

Be sure you avoid tucking your foot onto the knee joint of the opposite leg, as this puts too much pressure on the joint, and stand up straight so you don't overexert the back muscles.

If it's challenging for you to balance this move at first, hold your hands in front of you until you can properly stretch the upper body.

You can also tuck your foot behind your opposite ankle if you cannot bend and flex the muscles enough to keep it in proper position.

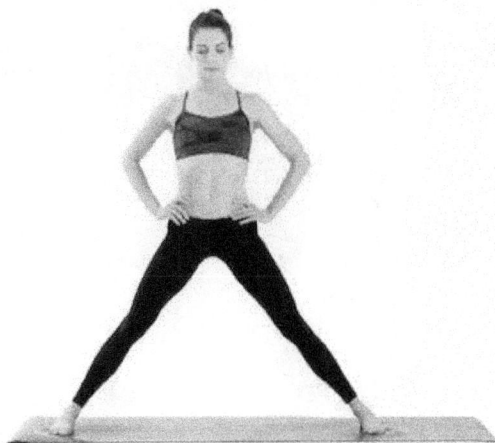

Wide Leg Stance

This movement strengthens and flexes the inner and outer muscles of the legs, and helps to keep you balanced.

As you perform this pose, feel your feet on the ground and work the muscles in the lower legs and feet themselves to keep you in place; don't tense the back muscles. This too will help support your posture during the pose, and even when your yoga routine is finished.

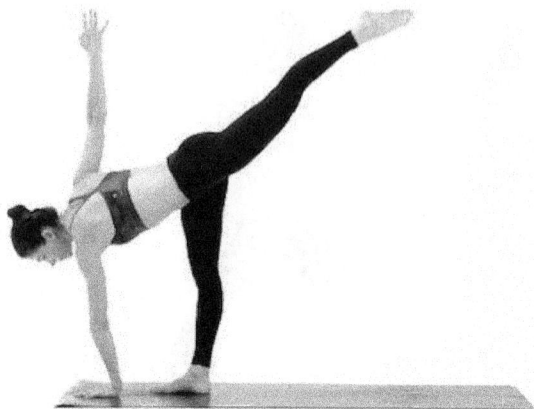

Half Moon Pose

This move stretches your entire back and the back of your extended leg, and the inside of the leg kept on the mat.

Keeping your one hand on the mat with the other outstretched to the side and behind you also opens up your entire chest, for better breathing. This also enables you to stay balanced in this pose.

Be sure you concentrate on your foot that's on the mat when in this pose, so you become aware of your balance.

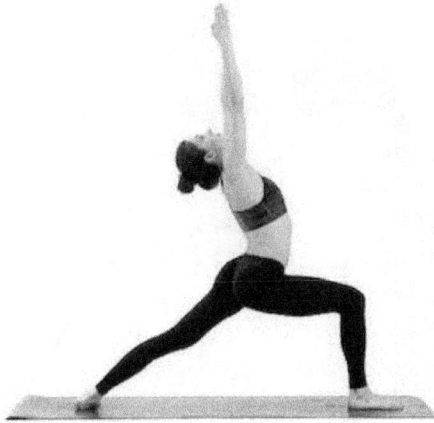

High Lunge Pose

This move strengthens and tones the buttocks and upper, back thighs. It also flexes the back and opens up the chest.

Note that the foot of the leg extended behind you should be turned outward, so it can better stretch all those muscles.

Lean back on the heel of the foot in front of you, for better balance and to keep your weight off your knees.

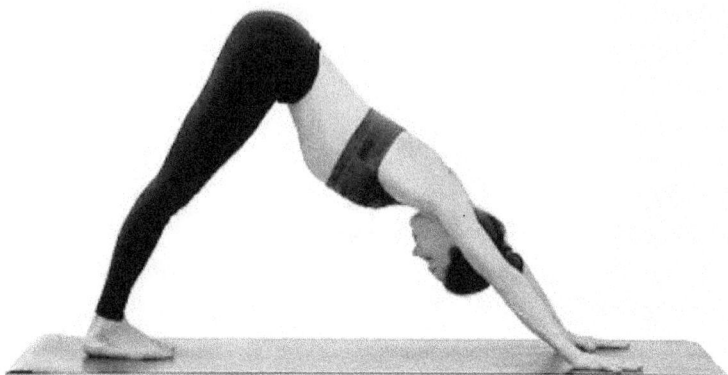

Downward Dog

This is one of the most basic and common yoga poses, and it's more beneficial than you may realize. For one thing, you can really tell how flexible your leg muscles are in this position, as you may not be able to flatten your feet very easily!

As your muscles get more flexible and supple, you'll find that you have better ability to keep your feet flat on the floor. This move also delivers more blood to the head, actually feeding and nourishing your brain!

Be sure to keep the back relaxed in this pose and do all your balancing with your leg muscles alone.

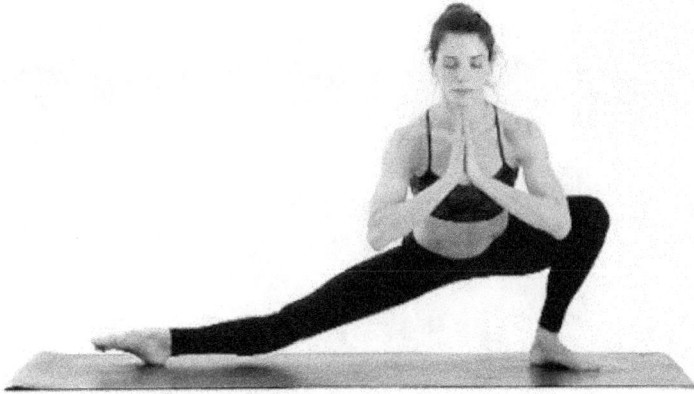

One Legged Squat

To perform this pose, start by standing up and then squat down, putting your hands on the floor in front of you for balance. Extend one leg to the side and lean back on both heels.

When you feel yourself balanced, pick up your hands and hold them in front of you. This move flexes all those inner thigh muscles that are hard to target with other moves.

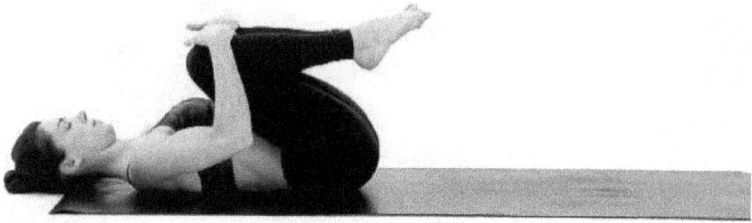

Knees to Chest

This move flexes the muscles of the legs and also helps strengthen the back.

When in this pose, concentrate on your back muscles and ensure they stay active; you shouldn't just collapse onto the mat.

When starting out, you may not be able to hug your legs very close to your chest, but focus each time you hold this pose on trying to stretch more deeply than before. Keep your hips planted on the mat so you don't stretch and injure the spine.

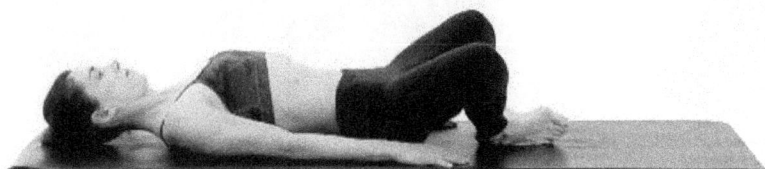

Reclined Goddess Pose

This position strengthens and tones those inner thigh muscles as well as the abdominals. Be sure you keep your back stretched so that you don't put all your weight on your lower back when in this position.

Pull your legs out as far as is comfortable, pushing them out further each time you try this pose.

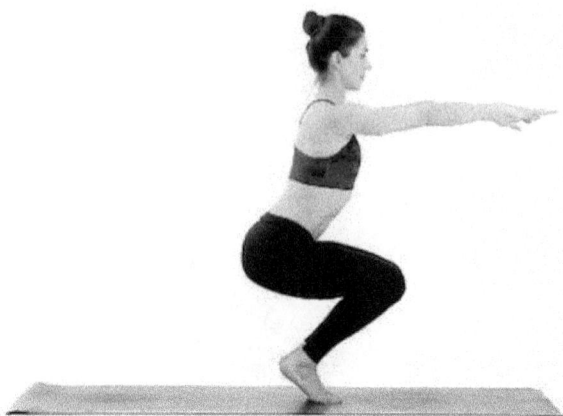

Awkward Pose

This pose is more than a basic squat; while you are on your toes, you don't want to lean forward and put weight on your knees. Instead, you are balancing yourself with your legs' muscles and buttocks alone, keeping them strengthened and firmed.

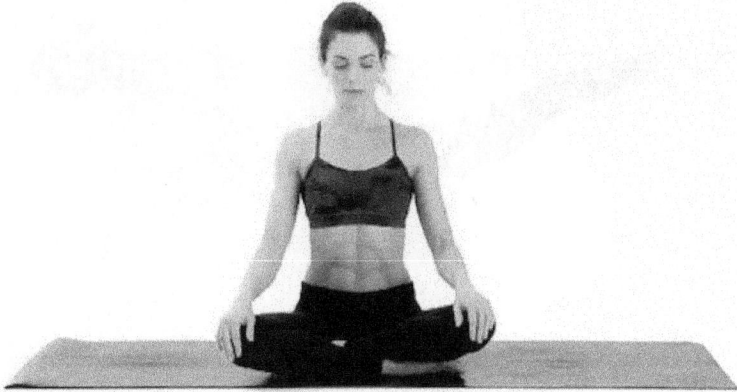

Easy Pose

Easy pose may seem pointless, but this is a good chance to note the alignment of your back and to feel your legs stretching.

This pose is also good for after a yoga routine, when you want to incorporate meditation or relaxation for stress reduction.

Between other poses, it can give your leg muscles or back muscles a rest so you don't overexert yourself, and ensure that you're not rushing through your yoga routine.

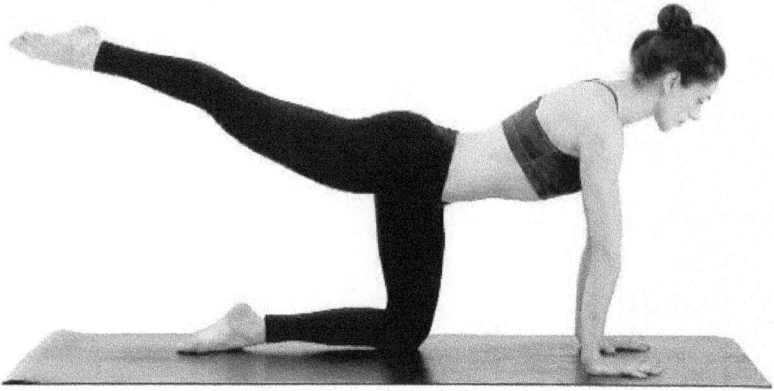

Half Table Pose

This pose flexes the buttocks and makes them firmed and toned. This also improves balance, as you learn to keep your weight supported even when on one leg.

Be sure you don't tense up the back muscles in this pose as this can cause undue stress, but keep the leg muscles firm and tight.

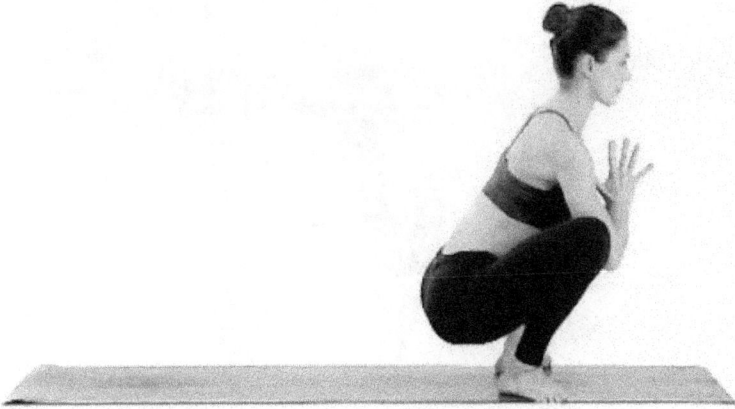

Wide Squat Pose

This pose strengthens the muscles and even the groin, which can aid in better digestion and easier elimination. It also teaches balance and makes you more aware to the muscles of the feet, helping to keep you upright.

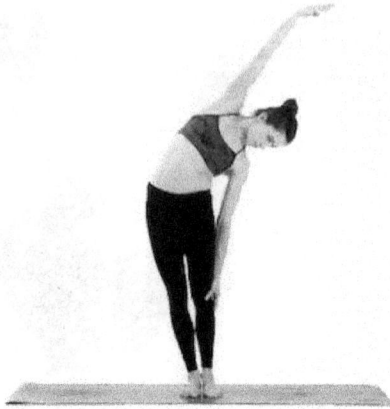

Standing Side Stretch

This pose not only stretches your sides but also keeps you balanced as you flex and keep the feet firm, to keep you in position.

Be sure you take a moment to feel your balance and be aware of your weight as it shifts when you perform this pose, and this will keep you balanced without falling over.

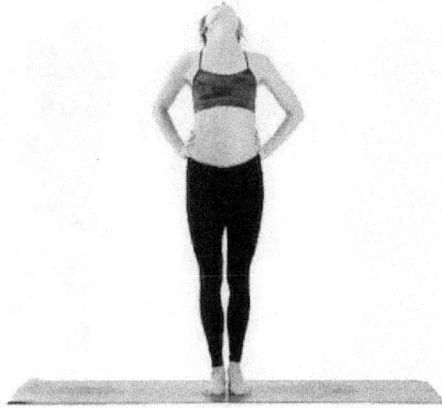

Standing Back Bend

This pose opens up the chest for better breathing and helps to alleviate pressure on the back muscles. You'll feel the muscles you've worked all day get stretched and may find you have less lower back pain when you use this pose.

This pose is good for use between other poses, as you flex and relax the back muscles and ensure they're not holding tension.

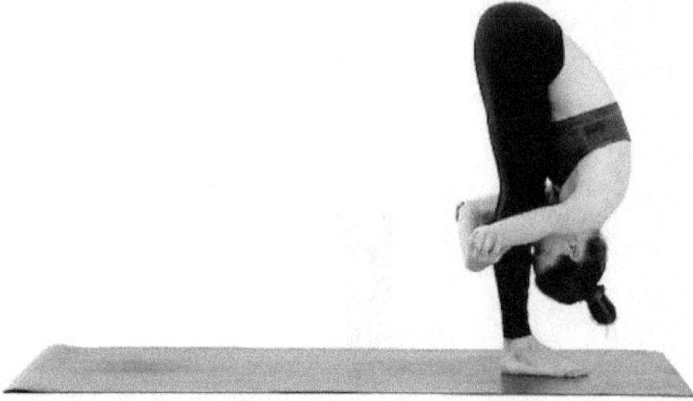

Standing Forward Bend

This pose is more challenging than you may realize, as you may tend to fall forward when in this pose, so you need to work those leg muscles to keep yourself balanced.

If the pose is too challenging, bend only as far as you can and keep your hands in front of your legs until those muscles get more flexible.

Be aware of your feet on the mat in this pose and feel them gripping the ground under you.

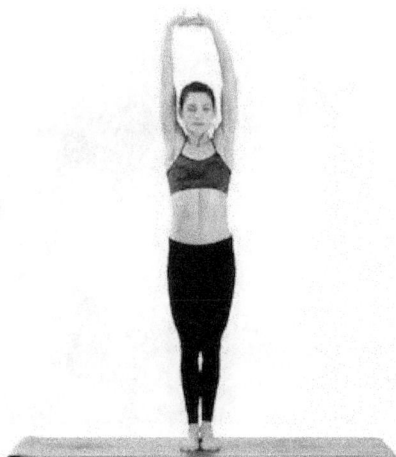

Palm Tree Pose

This pose may seem very basic, but pulling your arms up with your fingers clasped really stretches those side muscles. This also opens up your entire midsection so you can breathe better, and allows your lungs and liver to filter more toxins out of your body.

Breathing deeply during this pose relaxes you and prepares you for more challenging poses, and gives your body a rest between positions.

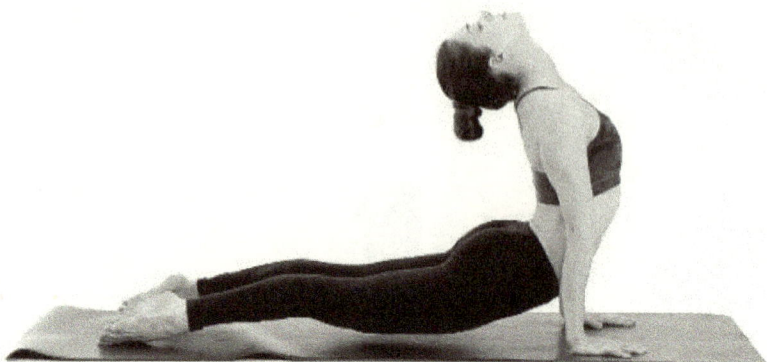

Cobra Pose

Note that your hips are off the ground in cobra pose, but the back is curved and not simply bent at the hips.

Curving the back into this position stretches them in the opposite direction than they normally face during the day, which then undoes stress on the back from sitting, standing, and poor posture.

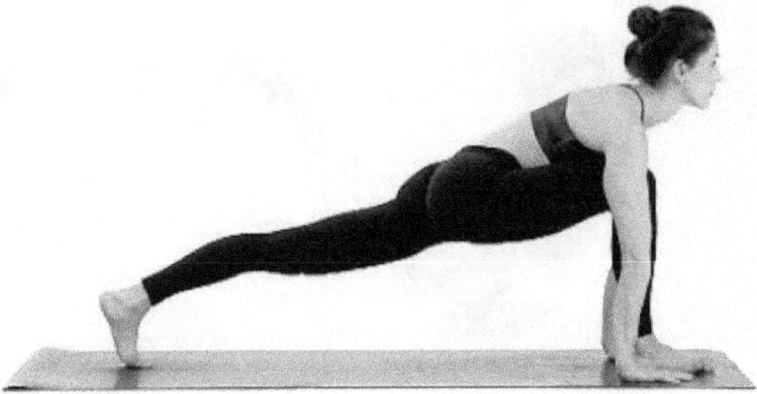

Runner's Lunge

While you are not resting your body entirely on your legs for this pose, the long stretch works those back muscles and buttocks. This also helps keep the knee joints flexible and active. Keep your hands on the mat so you're balanced in this pose.

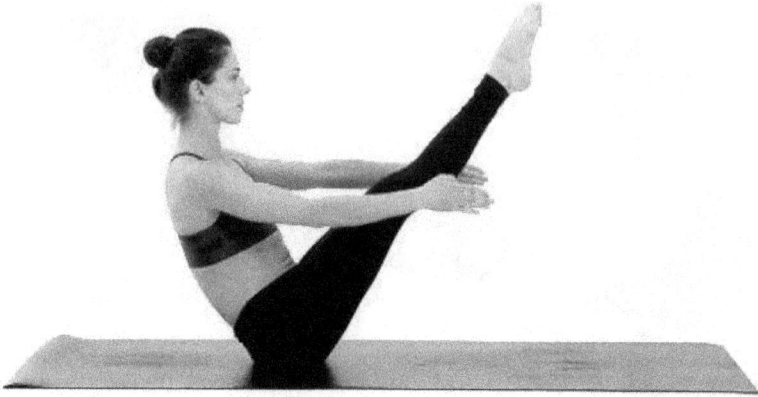

Boat Pose

To get into this position, start by sitting up, legs extended, hands on the floor. Lean your upper body back and then lift your legs up. Once balanced, lift your hands off the mat.

This position works the abdominals and back muscles, keeping your midsection strong.

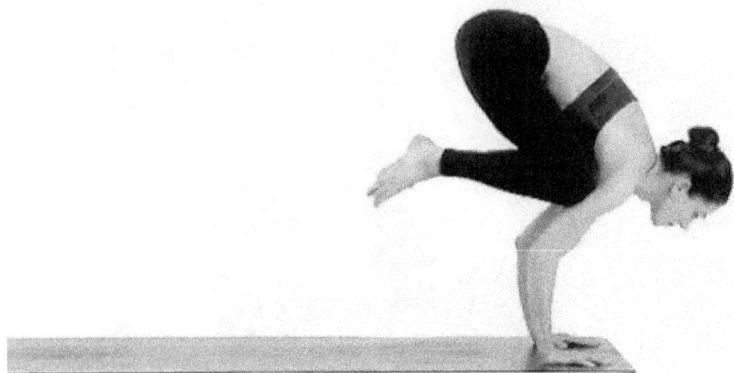

Crane Position

This position is difficult but it may not be as hard as you assume.

Get down on all fours and then put one knee onto that same arm, above the elbow. When you have your balance, lift the other knee into the same position. This may take some arm strength to hold for several seconds, but it helps build balance and flexibility all over your body.

Try it with your head against the wall when you first start out, for even more support.

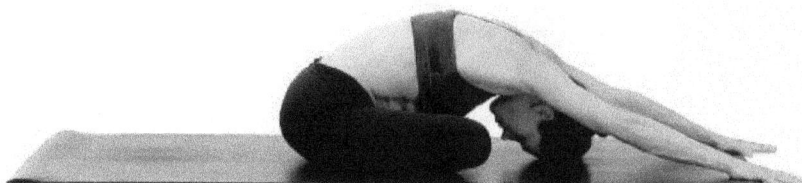

Easy Forward Bend

This position flexes the leg muscles, as you can see that they remain bent and crossed when you reach forward. The back and spine are also fully stretched. Be sure you hang your head and don't let your neck muscles stay tense during this move.

When starting out, simply reach as far forward as possible, and you'll eventually be able to stretch out completely in front of you.

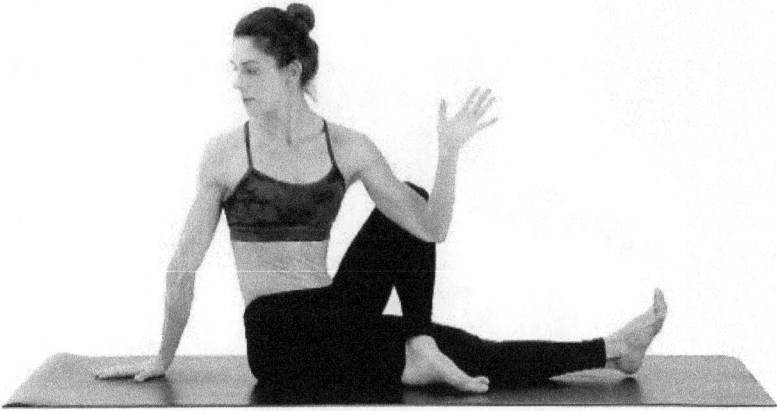

Half Spinal Twist

To get into this pose, gently guide your one leg into a bent position, with the foot over the opposite leg. Put one hand on the floor and gently twist at the waist, tucking the second arm over that corresponding leg for balance.

Guide the leg out of the pose when you change to the opposite side.

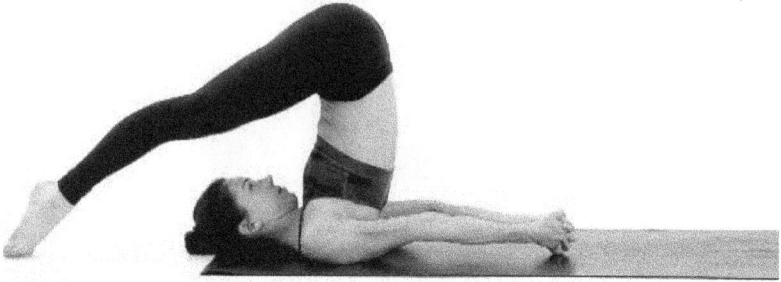

Plow Pose

This pose may take some work; start by lying on your back and reaching forward, over your toes, to stretch your back.

If you cannot lift and curve your back until your feet touch the floor behind you, simply stretch them as far as you can until your muscles become flexible enough to hold this pose.

You can also support your hips with your hands when first starting out, for easier balance.

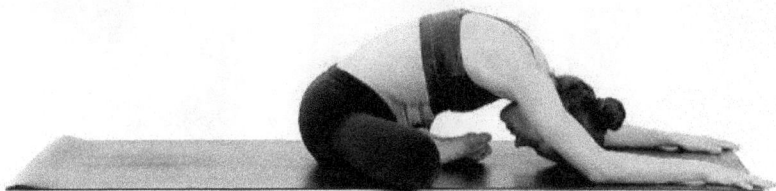

Cobbler Pose

This pose may be a bit advanced, as the legs are not crossed and the feet touch; this really stretches the leg muscles.

Note that the arms are outstretched but the elbows touch the mat, for added support. Be sure you don't overextend the back with this pose.

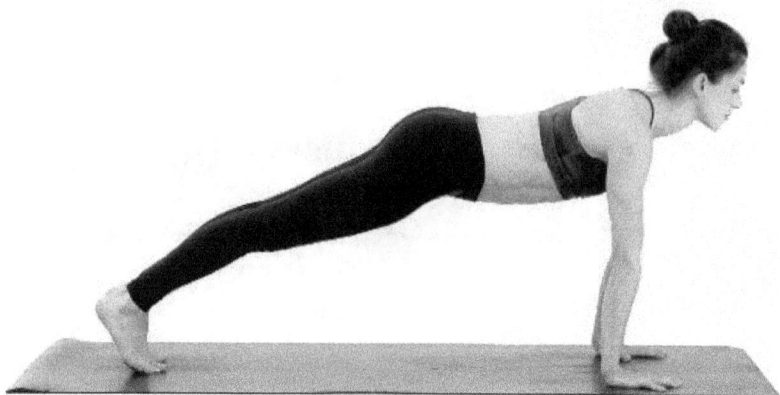

Plank Pose

This pose works the arm muscles and abdominals more than you may expect, as these muscles keep the body upright and supported.

Be sure the back is active but stretched and not carrying the weight of the body in this pose. Flex the leg muscles for added support as well. Try to keep your body aligned so that you don't curve the lower back either inward or outward.

Rest your head against a wall when first starting this move, for more support.

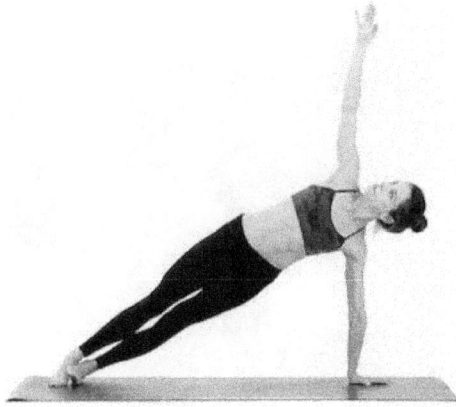

Side Plank Pose

To begin this pose, get into a plank position, both arms and feet on the ground, as if doing a pushup. Gently shift your weight to one arm and leg and then twist the opposite arm up and over your body. Keep both feet on the ground, to disperse your weight and keep you balanced.

Note your alignment in this pose as you don't want to push your lower back out or let your stomach collapse in front of you. Be sure you're pushing up with your arm muscles and not putting pressure on your elbow.

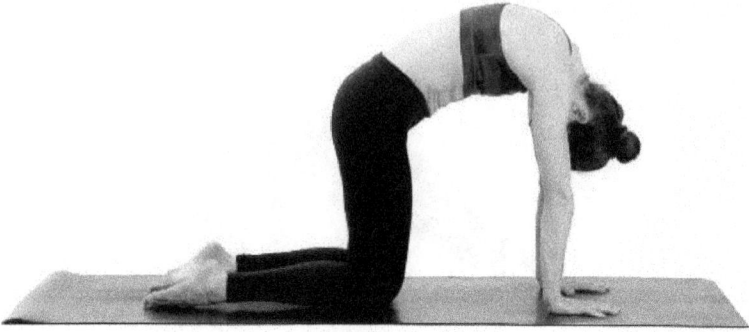

Cat Pose

This pose stretches and flexes the back muscles and loosens the neck. Start on your hands and knees and then gently curve the middle of the back up, pulling in the buttocks slightly.

Don't tense or hold the muscles, but simply feel this stretch along your back.

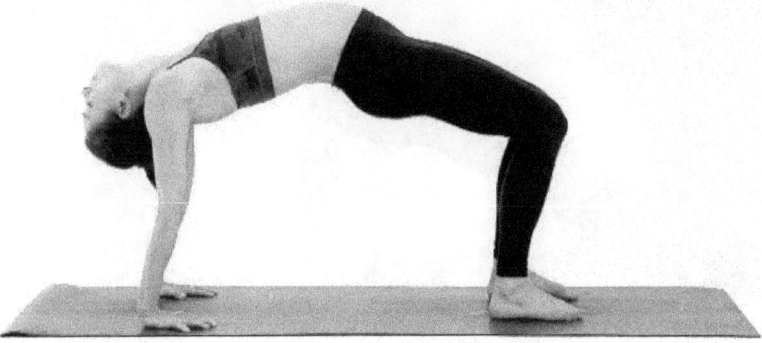

Crab Pose

This difficult pose is actually easier to achieve than you think!

Sit on the floor and extend your legs in front of you. Reach your hands behind you and shift your weight to your feet and hands as you lift your legs and buttocks off the ground. Be sure to curve gently into and out of this position, so you don't injure your back.

Feel your leg muscles work and your buttocks staying tense to keep you in place and keep you supported; don't let your back to any of the lifting and holding in this position.

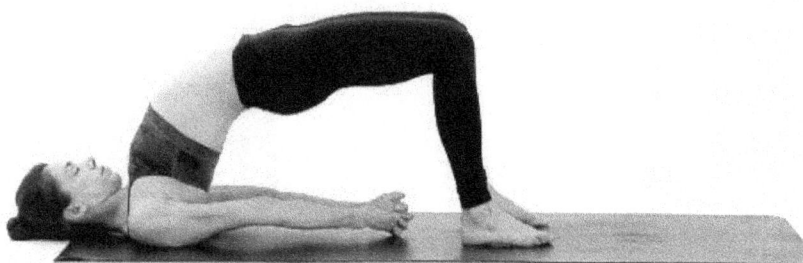

Bridge Pose

When holding bridge pose, you want to ensure you are using your shoulders and upper body to support your weight, and that you keep your feet on the floor, your leg muscles active. This will ensure you don't put undue stress on the neck muscles and damage any ligaments in the neck area.

When pushing up into bridge pose, be sure you push with your heels and not your knees.

Otherwise, you may tear ligaments in your knees and may not work the buttocks and upper leg muscles. Flex the abdominals so they stay active and your stomach muscles get a good workout.

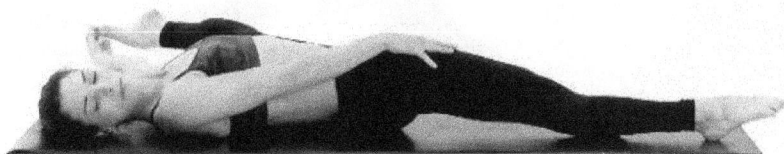

Extended Hand to Foot Pose

If you have a hard time extending your leg straight out when getting into this pose, move it into a ninety-degree angle as far as it will go, and then use your hand to help move it even further toward your head.

Keep your leg straight and don't bend the knee or put undue pressure on the back. Your opposite leg should stay active and help to balance your body.

You also want to ensure you don't simply collapse the back, as this can put pressure on your midsection and cause damage to the spine.

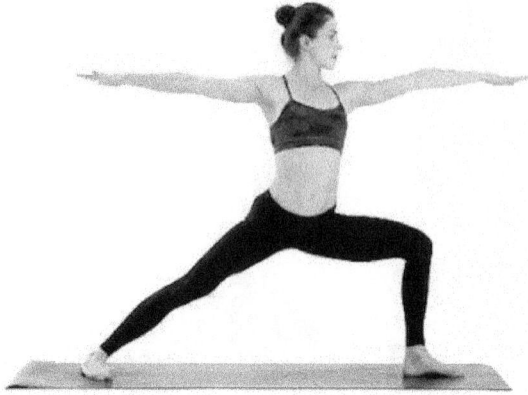

Warrior II Pose

Warrior II is a good way to improve balance and coordination and your overall flexibility.

To achieve this pose, step out to one side and gain your balance, and then put your arms out, gently twisting at the waist to the side opposite your outstretched leg.

Be sure your legs are holding you upright and you're not putting stress on your back or neck. Your leg should also be outstretched enough that you have proper alignment and form, and aren't resting on your knees.

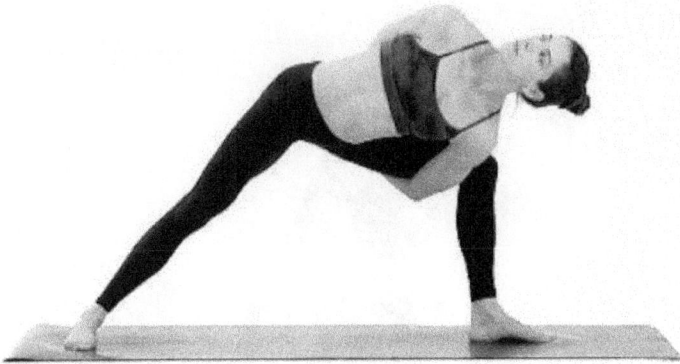

Side Angle Pose

To perform this pose, you want to stand straight and then put one leg out to the side.

Gain your balance, and lean slightly over the leg that is still planted. Feel your feet gripping the mat. Wrap your arms around that planted leg. Your arms shouldn't be stretched but are just letting your legs do the work in keeping you upright.

You should also feel your abdominals tighten and tense up in this position, as they will also keep you in place.

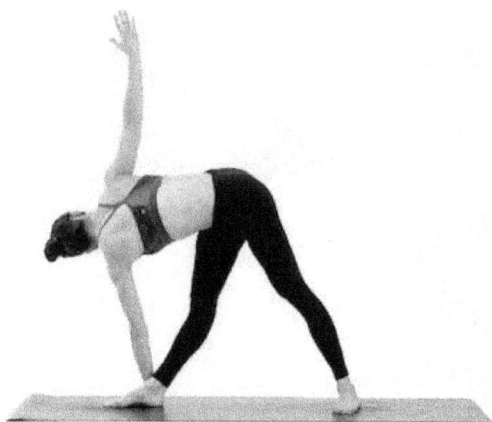

Tucked Triangle Pose

This pose is actually more challenging than it looks, as it's difficult to stay balanced when your feet are spread and your body is twisted.

Start in a stance with feet shoulder-width apart, arms outstretched. Twist at the waist and reach one arm over the opposite foot. Be sure to keep the other arm outstretched behind you, so you form this triangle.

If you tend to fall out of this pose when you first begin, put that hand in front of the foot, not behind it, flat on the mat. Work on keeping your balance between your feet and remember to have your leg muscles hold you in place, not your knees or back.

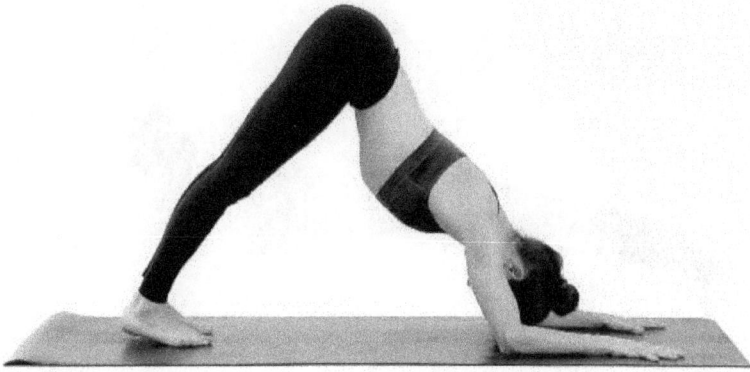

Dolphin Pose

This bend is a bit different than others as lowering your upper body so your arms rest on the mat really stretches those back-leg muscles.

In this pose, be sure you're not flexing and holding the back tense, as it shouldn't be working to support your weight.

If you can't flatten your feet, simply stretch your legs as far as they will go and then you can work into a longer stretch over time. Keep your head down as well, so you're not putting undue stress on the neck and shoulders.

Also, remember that poses like these aren't good for use after a heavy meal, as stomach acids may then move into the esophagus, so be careful of this pose for a routine after dinnertime.

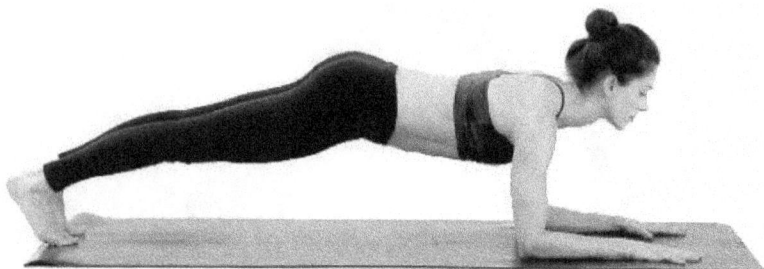

Dolphin Plank

This pose is a bit easier than a standard plank pose because you're resting your arms on the mat, so your weight is more readily dispersed. It still works the abdominals and back muscles, but be sure you don't hold any of these muscles tense. You also want to keep your neck relaxed and flexible and not tense.

If the position becomes difficult, lean forward with your toes just slightly, so your weight it pushed onto your arms and not your legs and toes, and not your stomach. Be sure you feel your flat palms on the mat, holding you steady.

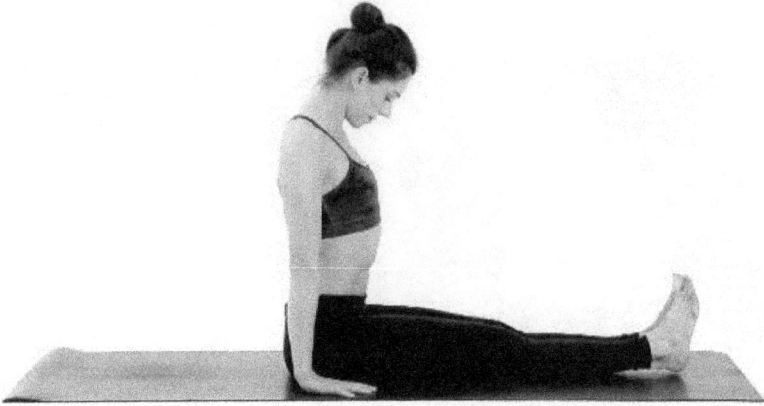

Staff Pose

Staff pose is not just about sitting, but is a chance for your body to get a break between tougher poses and for you to tune into your posture and leg muscles. Sitting up straight also allows you to breathe more freely.

Note how the ankles are just slightly elevated; this keeps the leg muscles active and flexed. Pull the belly in also, not allowing it to simply collapse in front of you. This will ensure you can breathe deeply and are holding your posture upright.

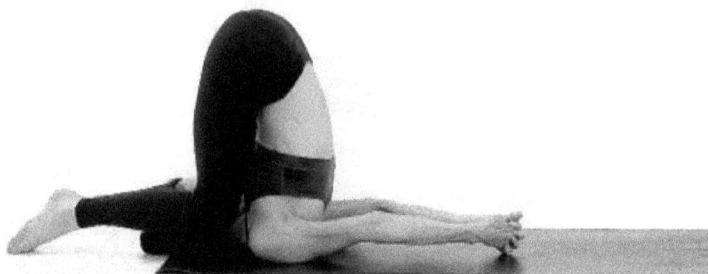

Ear Pressure Pose

This pose can be difficult, but it helps to guide your legs behind your head with your hands on your hips, giving your body added support. Use a pillow or foam block under your head so your legs don't need to actually reach the floor to support you.

If you cannot reach the floor with your knees, hold them with your hands rather than putting your arms out behind you, or put your hands on the mat and give your body support.

Note that the feet are on the floor, behind your head, which also helps with support.

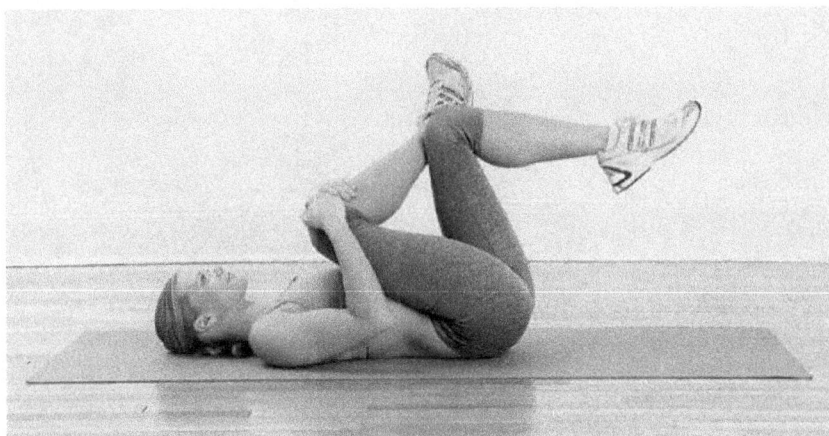

Reclined Cross-Legged Pose

This pose gives your legs a deep stretch while also keeping the knee joints flexible and fluid. Note that the hips and buttocks are pulled off the floor just slightly; this will ensure a nice stretch of the spine.

Be sure the back is active and doesn't just collapse onto the mat under you. The belly should also be flexed and tense, helping you stay in position.

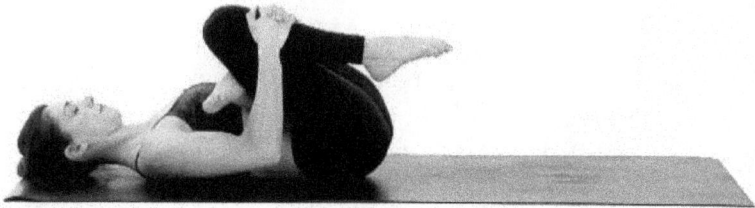

Reclined Pigeon Pose

This pose is similar to Knees to Chest, but note that one leg is bent in front of the body. This allows for a much deeper stretch of the hamstring and all the muscles of the thighs and buttocks.

Be sure you keep the neck relaxed in this pose and not tense, so you don't pull those muscles or put pressure on the shoulders.

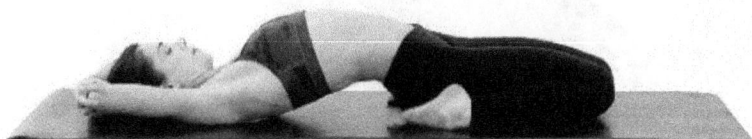

Reclined Hero Pose

This pose gives a tremendous stretch to the hamstrings and all the muscles of the legs and back.

If you cannot fully recline, lean as far back as you can, keeping your body aligned and your hands behind you. You can also start this pose in a reclined position and tuck your legs back as far as they will go.

You should feel a deeper stretch with each time you get into this position.

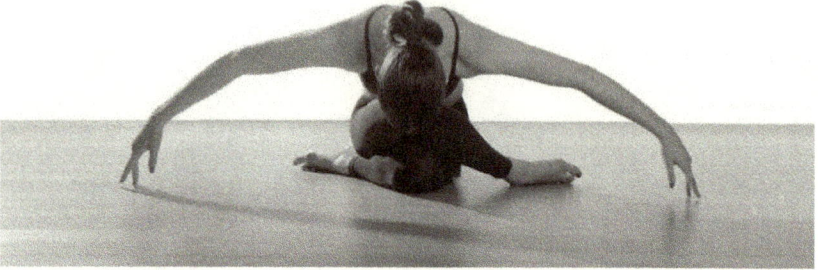

Dragon Pose

This pose stretches the legs and back muscles and keeps the upper body open for better breathing.

Note that the fingertips are touching the mat, for added balance. The head should also be curved downward and not facing up, so the neck is not holding tension.

If you cannot cross your legs this deeply for this pose, allow your top leg a bit more space and don't tuck it so close to your body. Curve your back as far as you can go to reach this pose.

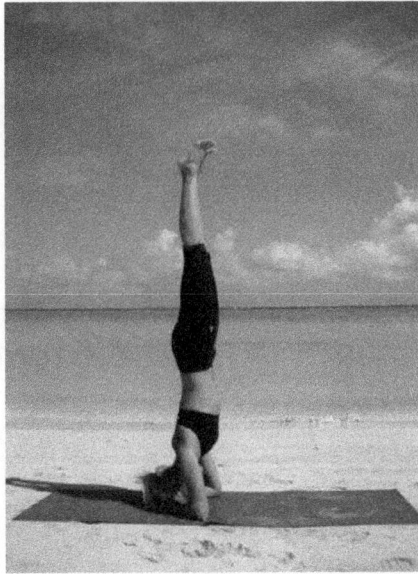

Headstand

A headstand is a very basic pose, allowing for better blood flow to the brain and upper body.

However, it can be difficult for adults to do a headstand, as it takes a tremendous amount of balance and coordination. You might have a friend help you get into this position, and use a wall to lean against for better balance.

You can also walk yourself into a headstand rather than simply trying to flip your body over; put your upper arms on the mat and then your legs on your arms, then lift one leg in the air, leaning against a wall, then lift the other leg into position.

Be sure you're not putting undue pressure on the head and neck in this position and that you keep your body in alignment.

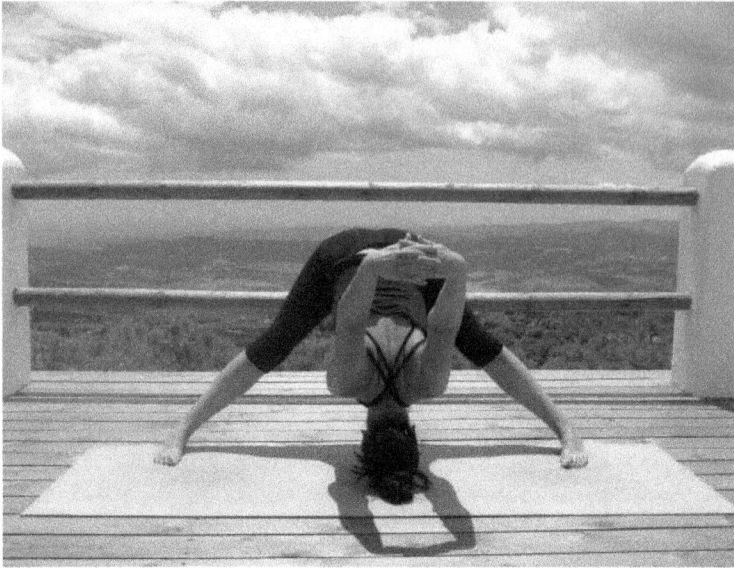

Dragon II Pose

Gently rest your head on the mat for this pose but don't put weight on the head or shoulders.

If you cannot stretch your arms up and behind you this far, simply hold them outstretched to your sides for added balance. Let your leg muscles hold you up rather than your back.

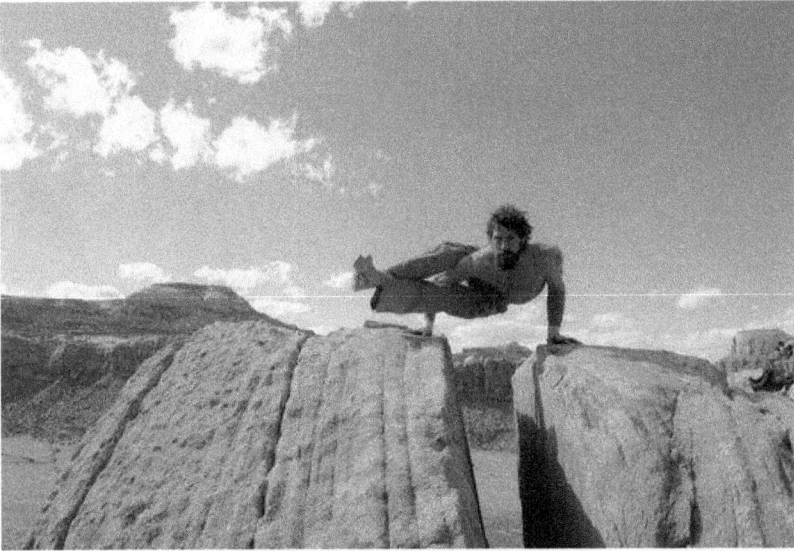

Eight Angle Pose

For advanced yogis, this is a pose you can work up to as you practice your yoga routine.

On your side, put your dominant arm through your legs and flatten your hands on the mat. Note that the top leg is bent slightly, to allow room for the arm. Push yourself up, lifting your legs but keeping your feet on the mat for balance.

Once you've established your position, lift your legs off the mat entirely.

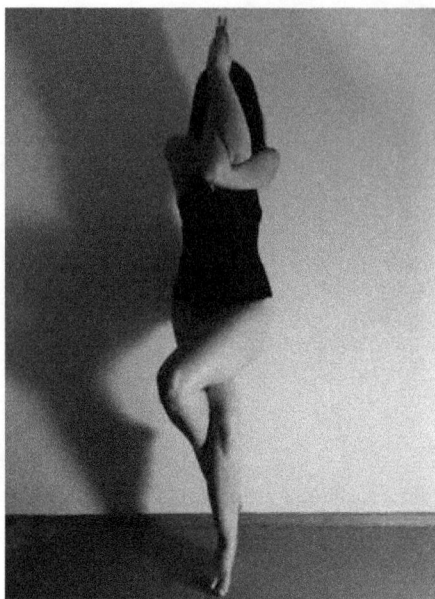

Eagle Pose

This pose is very good for balance and coordination, as wrapping your arms together forces you to rely only on your one leg for support. Advanced yogis may crouch or squat down more, which also stretches and flexes those leg muscles.

Be sure you're not leaning forward and putting pressure on the back for eagle pose, but rely only on the legs for balance.

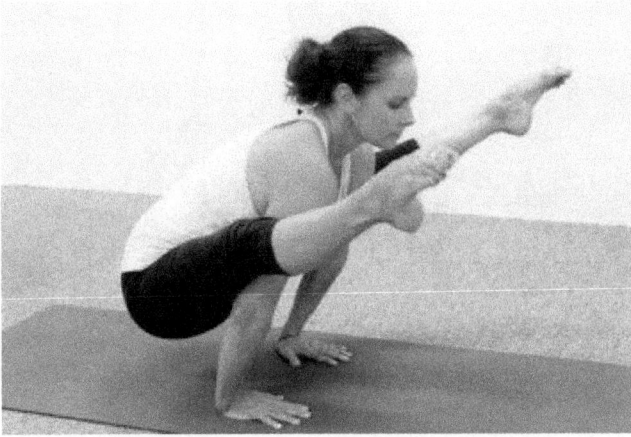

Firefly Pose

This advanced pose teaches balance of the arms and upper body while stretching the groin and legs.

Start with your legs outstretched and put your arms between them, flat on the mat. Push up with your toes so you lift your buttocks off the floor, then your lower legs.

When you have your balance, you can lift your feet off the floor as well.

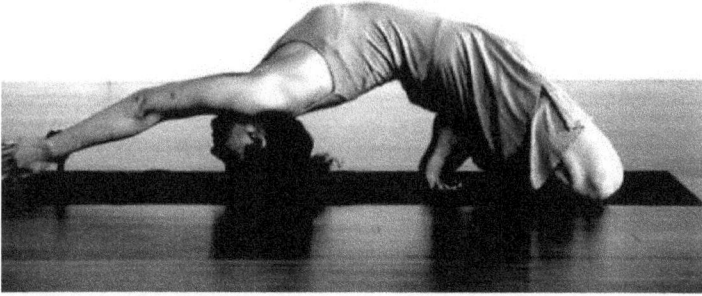

Fish Pose

To make this pose easier for you, walk your arms behind you while keeping your hands on the mat, rather than trying to simply lean back with your arms in the air.

Be sure you curve your back into this pose and don't just bend at the waist, so you don't put pressure on the lower back.

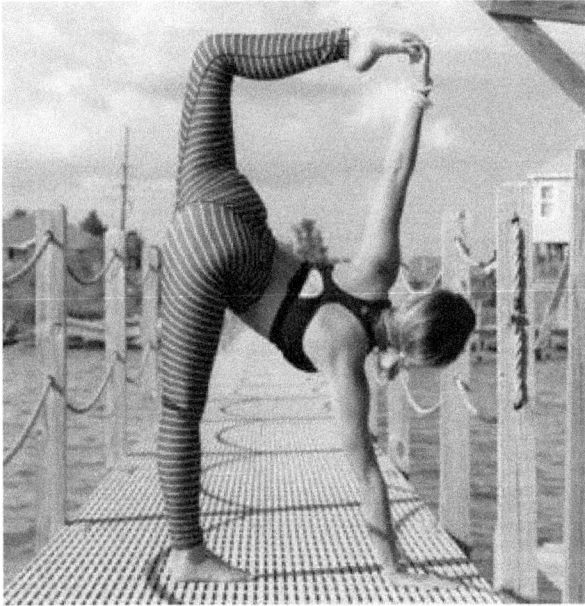

Half Moon Pose

To perform this pose, stand with feet shoulder width apart and then bend to one side, lifting your opposite leg and putting that hand on the mat. Bend your lifted leg at the knee and reach for it with your open hand.

Be sure your weight is on your hand that is on the mat so you can keep your balance. Lean back on your heel of the foot that is planted so you don't put pressure on the knees.

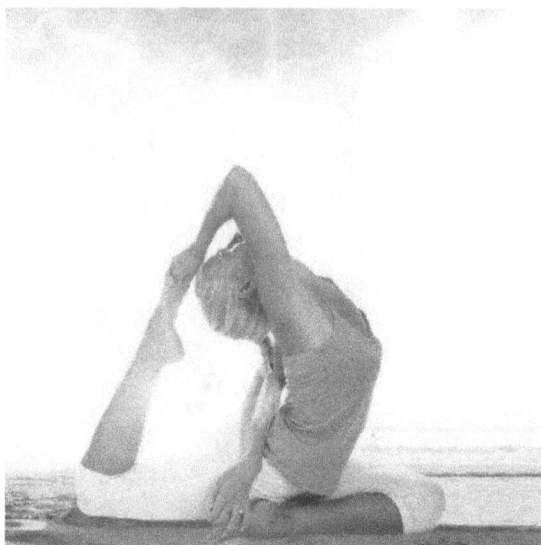

King Pigeon I Pose

This pose may be a bit advanced, but start by crossing your left leg in front of you, and then gently guide your right leg behind you. Bend your right knee and reach up and over with your right hand to help your leg bend.

If you cannot bend the right knee, keep the leg behind you so it gets a good stretch and work up to this pose over time.

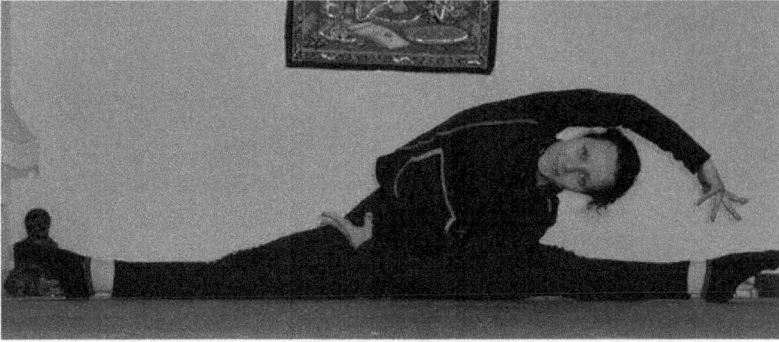

Monkey Pose

To perform the splits, start with your legs outstretched and to your sides as far as they will go, and then guide them even further with your hands, as far as is comfortable.

Keep your left hand on the mat in front of you and gently stretch to the left, lifting your right arm up and over. Be sure your upper body is curved and not just bent at the waist. Gently twist out of this position and then bend to the other side.

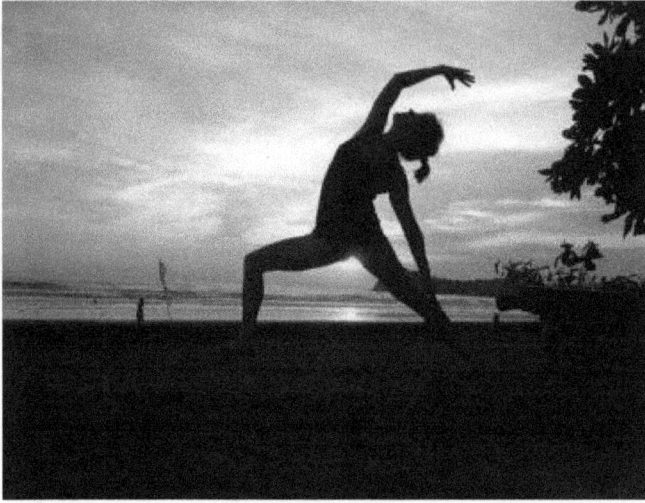

Warrior Pose

When in warrior pose, be sure your weight is on the heel of the planted foot and not the knee.

Flex the muscles of the leg that is outstretched so they hold you upright. Bend gently into a curve over that leg, reaching that arm down the leg while curving the other arm over the body.

Be sure the neck is also curved and not bent so you don't pull on the neck muscles.

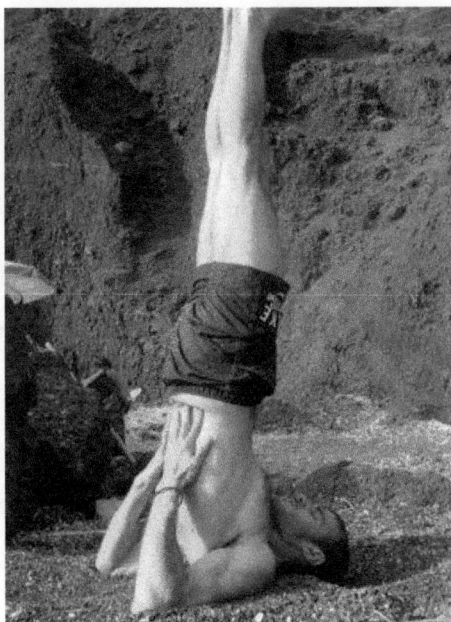

Shoulder Stand

To perform a shoulder stand, get close to a wall and walk your legs up until you're in position. Hold your hips with your hands to keep yourself balanced.

Once you're stronger, you can get into this position without the wall.

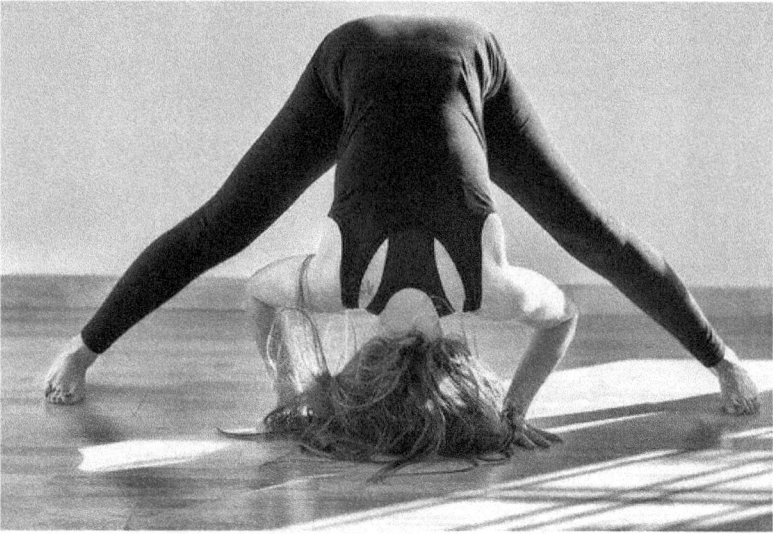

Wide Legged Forward Bend

To safely perform this position, curve your body forward; don't simply bend at the waist. Keep your hands flat on the mat so you can be balanced and steady.

Your head should also be flat on the mat so you increase blood flow to the brain and don't pull muscles in the neck.

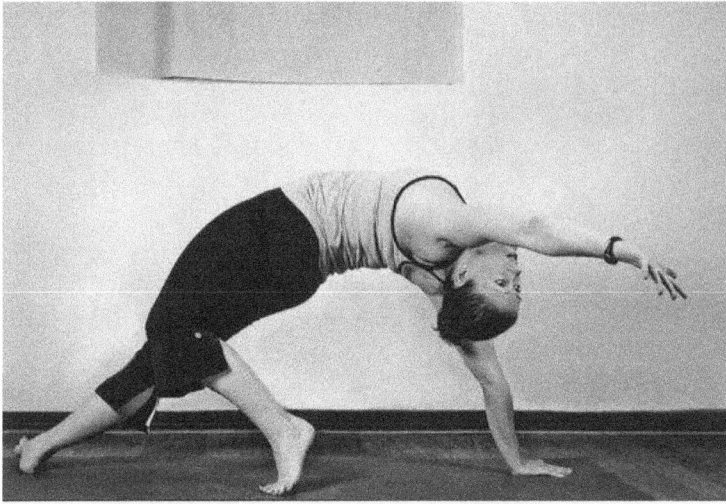

Wild Thing Pose

To get into wild thing pose, stand with your feet shoulder width apart, then gently lower yourself to the ground so your hands are flat on the mat.

Bend and curve your body backward while walking your hands back behind you. Keep your right hand flat, as you see in the photo, and step your right leg out, gently lifting your left hand behind you.

Be sure your neck is gently curved and not straight so you don't pull those muscles, and balance your left leg so it holds your weight and you don't put pressure on the knee.

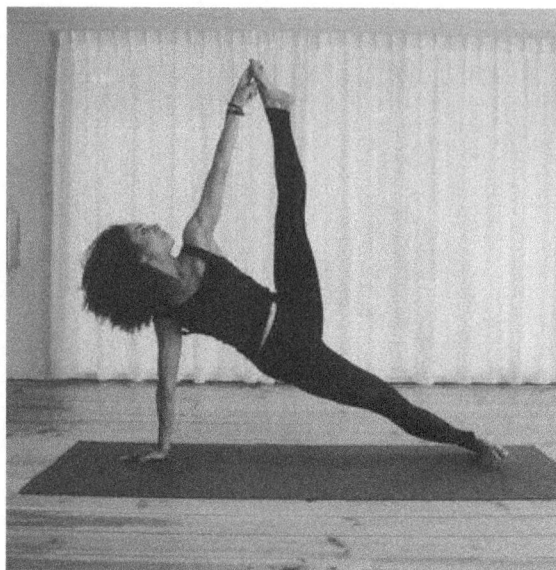

Side Plank Pose with Leg Lift

This side plank pose is more challenging than other plank poses.

Get into side plank and then gently bend your upper leg at the knee, then hold the foot with your corresponding hand and guide the leg straight up.

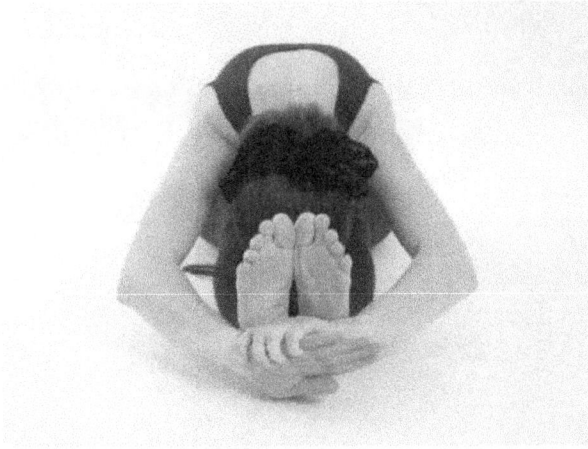

Seated Forward Bend

This position may be more challenging than you realize, but it keeps the leg muscles active while allowing them a break from supporting your body weight.

Be very sure you curve your body forward rather than just bending at the waist, to alleviate pressure off the lower back.

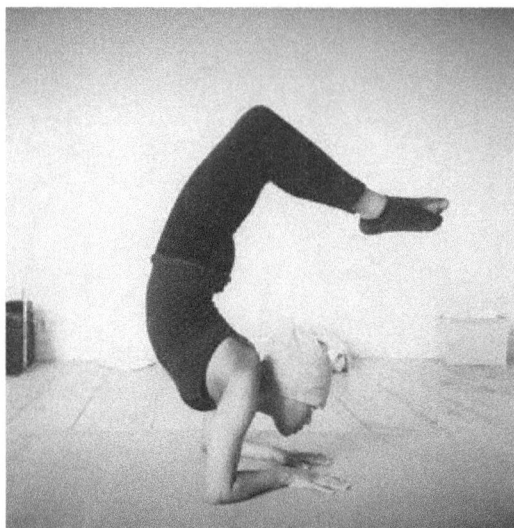

Scorpion Pose

You might have a friend help you get into this position your first few times trying it.

Keep your head on the ground as you lift your legs, then push yourself up with your arms as you curve your legs behind you. Keep the legs muscles active so they support your weight.

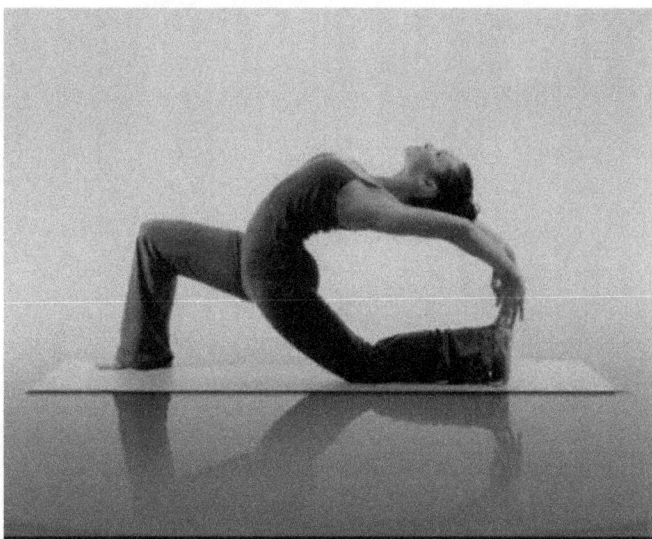

Low Lunge Pose

Start with a lunge and lower your back leg to the mat. Curve your back up and around, gently reaching your arms up and then behind you.

Don't put too much pressure on your back or knees but allow your planted foot to hold your weight instead.

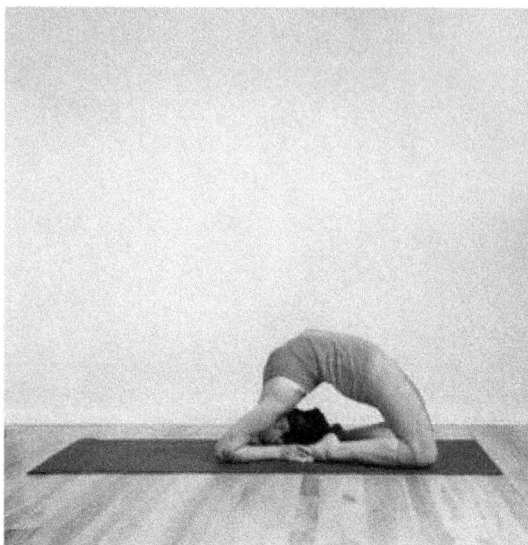

King Pigeon II Pose

Gently walk your hands behind you to get into this pose rather than simply trying to bend.

If you cannot curve your head all the way down to the mat, do the best you can and get into the deepest curve, without putting pressure on your back. Let your hands help to support your weight overall.

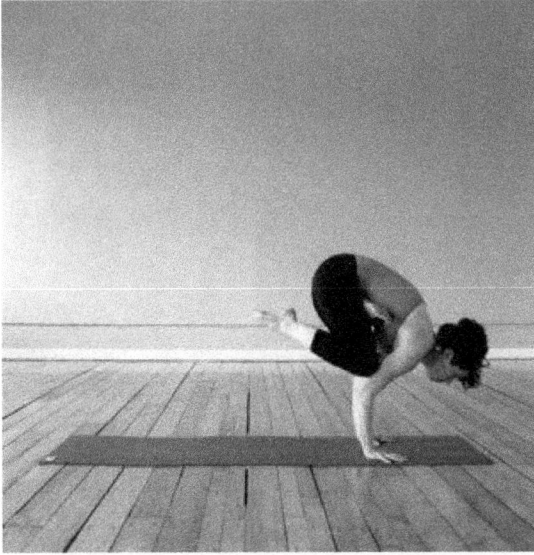

Half Lotus Crow Pose

It's good to lean forward on your head and hands while you cross your leg in front of the other when getting into this position. Feel your balance on your hands and arms and then push yourself up, but don't push with your neck.

Remember to lean your leg onto your upper arm and not the elbow joint in this position.

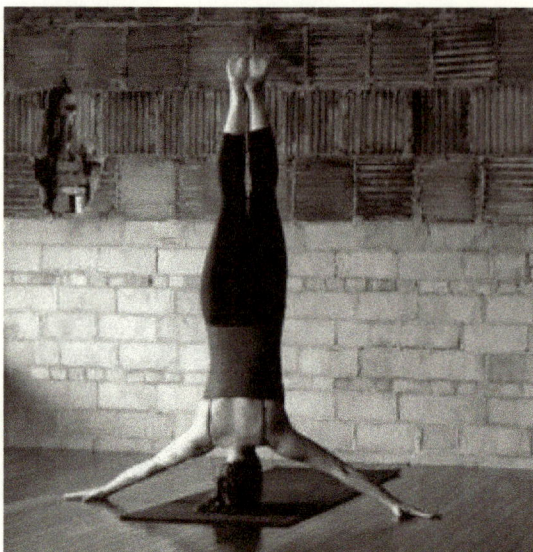

Iron Cross Headstand

Don't put pressure on the head and neck in this pose, but keep your palms flat on the mat to balance your weight. It's good to put your hands in this position before getting into the headstand so your weight is always dispersed and you won't aggravate the neck.

Start by leaning against a wall if this pose is too challenging, or have a friend help you get into the pose.

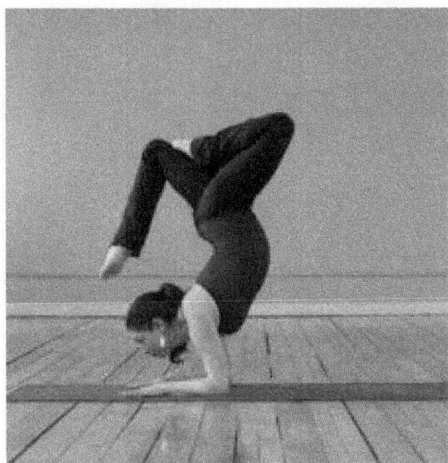

Scorpion with Broken Tail

This position is easiest to achieve if you put your left leg behind your right before pushing up with your arms into a handstand, and then curving your legs up and over your head. You can use the tucked leg to help push yourself into position.

Keep your upper arms flat on the mat so they provide the most support, or have a friend help you into this position as needed.

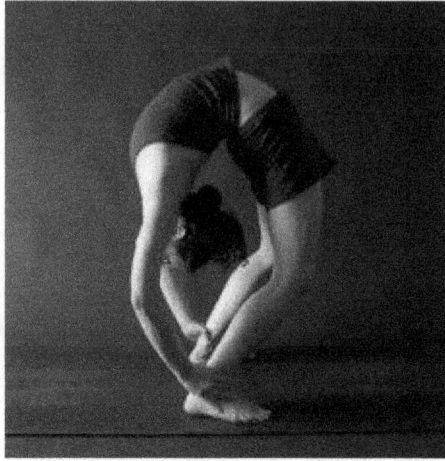

Standing Bound Pose

This is not a simple back stretch, but this pose allows all the legs of the muscles to curve and stretch while still keeping you balanced and flexed.

Holding your ankles allows for more control and alleviates some tension in the legs. You can actually reach behind you and hold your ankles and then push your body up and into the curve, rather than trying to curve backwards from a standing position.

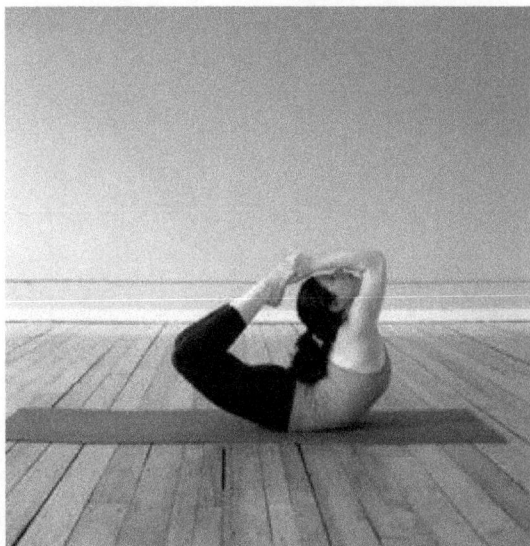

Toe Bow Pose

Grasp your toes while in a reclined position and use your hands to pull your legs up and off the mat. Gently curve your back into this position at the same time.

Be sure to keep your stomach muscles active so they give you full support.

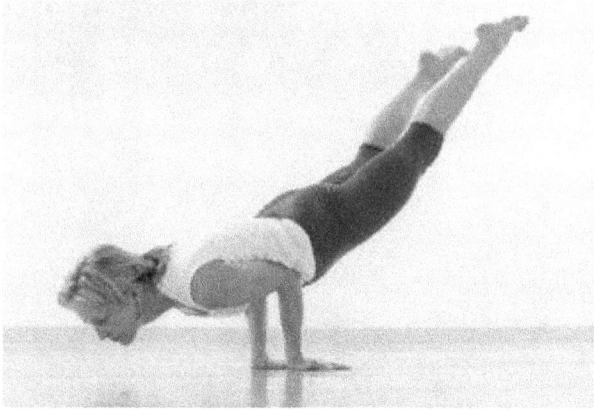

Peacock Pose

Use a wall for support when first trying this pose; put your feet on the wall and walk upward as you rest on your hands, then pull your feet away by leaning forward so you become accustomed to your arms supporting you.

Turning the palms inward also puts more pressure on the base of the hand, which is stronger than the fingertips.

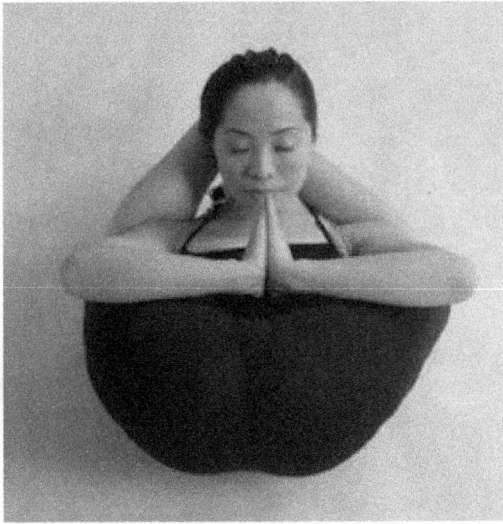

Sleeping Yogi Pose

This pose may look odd but it helps to stretch the digestive muscle and may allow for easier elimination.

Gently curve forward from an inclined position in this pose and then guide the legs behind the head with your hands.

If you cannot hold the entire pose, push the legs up and back as far as possible and hold them with your hands.

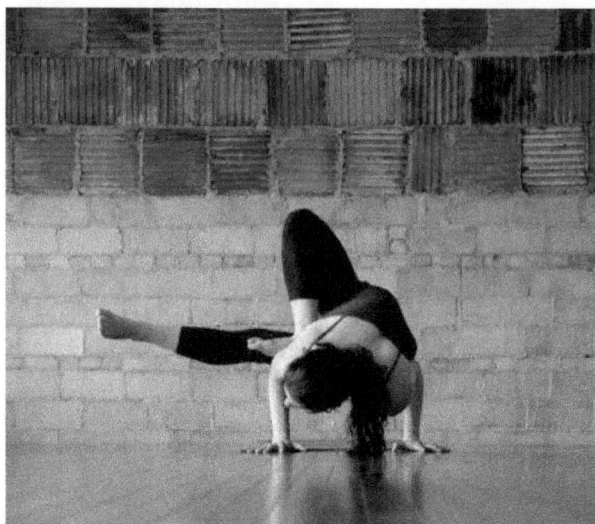

Hummingbird

Keep your head on the mat while you come into a handstand with this pose and then push one leg across the body, resting the opposite leg on that thigh.

Try this against the wall when starting out, or have a friend hold you in this position.

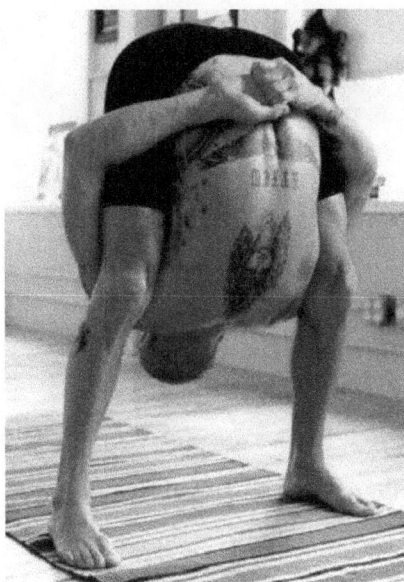

Firefly II

Notice the curve on the back of this pose; bend forward and then reach your hands to your buttocks and push yourself into a deeper curve. Holding the hands will allow for more support.

If you cannot curve this deeply then just hold your hands as far as they can reach behind your back.

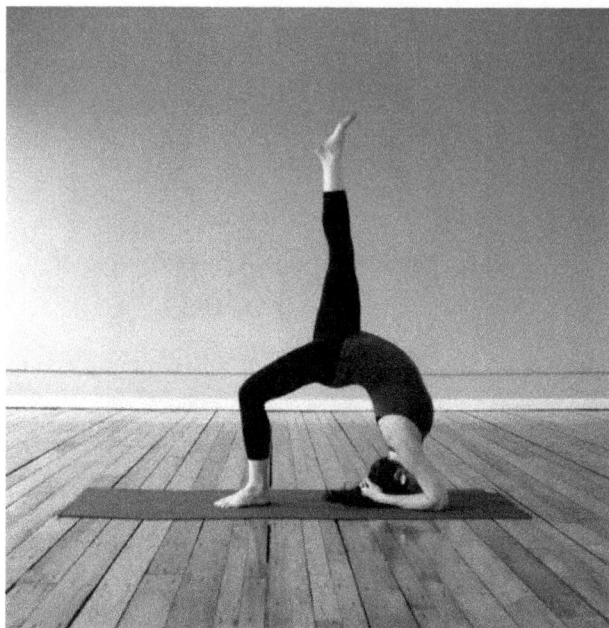

One-Legged Staff

Start with your hands on the mat and your body curved backwards, then lift one leg in the air. Once you have your balance, lower your arms so you're only supported by your planted foot and upper arm.

Don't put pressure on your head and neck in this position but stretch the raised leg as far as possible.

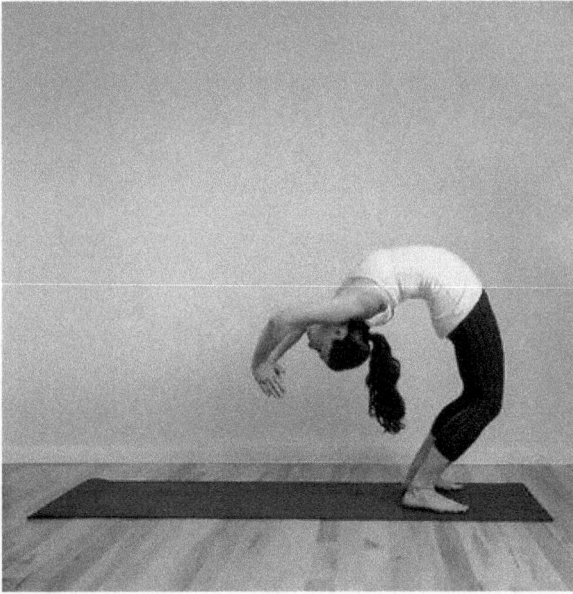

Drop Back

To reach this position, gently curve your back and reach your arms behind you as far as they will go. Bring them together while feeling your feet on the mat, planted and firm. Your thighs should also be working to keep you in place and balanced.

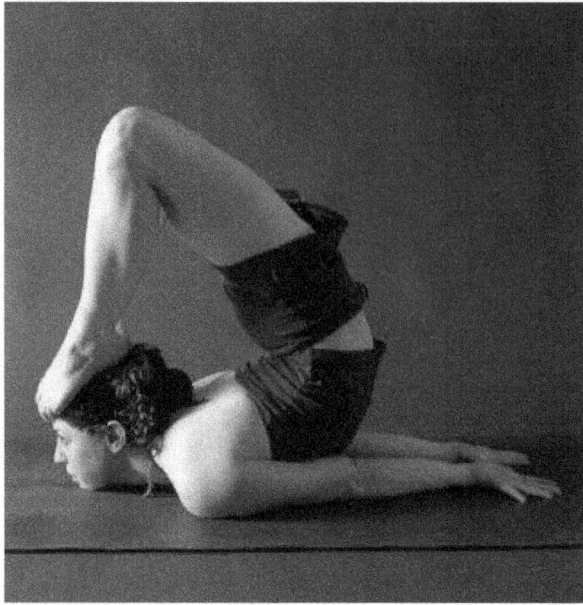

Locust Scorpion

Use your arms to gently guide your legs into position for this pose. If you cannot reach the top of your head, just hold your legs up as far as they will go into this curve. Putting your hands on the mat behind you will help to keep you balanced.

You might also have a friend help to guide your legs into the pose, holding you in place and keeping you balanced.

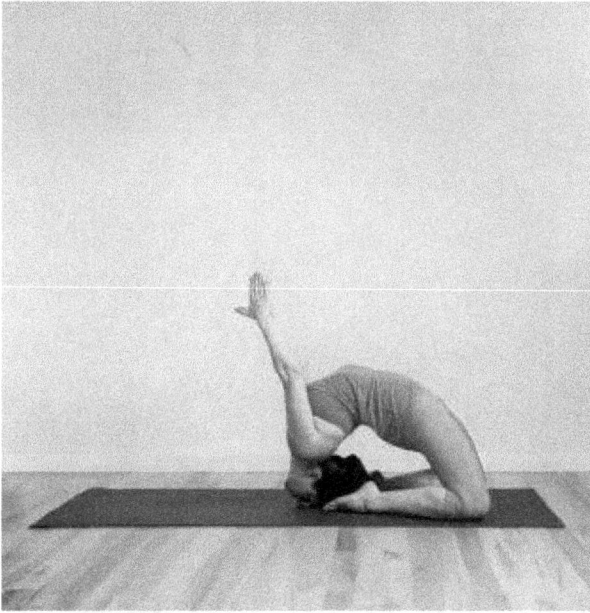

Thunderbolt

Keep your hands on the mat while you bend your back into a curve so you can remain supported as you get into this pose. Once you feel comfortable with your head on your feet, reach in front of you while flexing your leg muscles to keep yourself in place.

If the curve is too deep, simply reach back as far as you can and keep your arms in front of you to add to your overall balance.

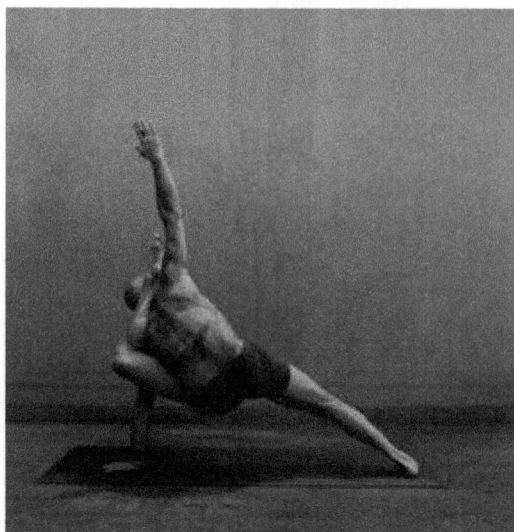

Leg Behind the Head Sage Pose

This is a very advanced pose but a good one to work up to in your routine.

When you can bend one leg back behind your body, tuck it around your back or shoulders if you can reach that far. Keep your buttocks on the mat to provide balance and the push up with that same hand and the opposite leg. Once you're into position, reach into the air with the opposite arm.

You can also try this position with a foam block under you for added support until you can flex enough to keep yourself in the air.

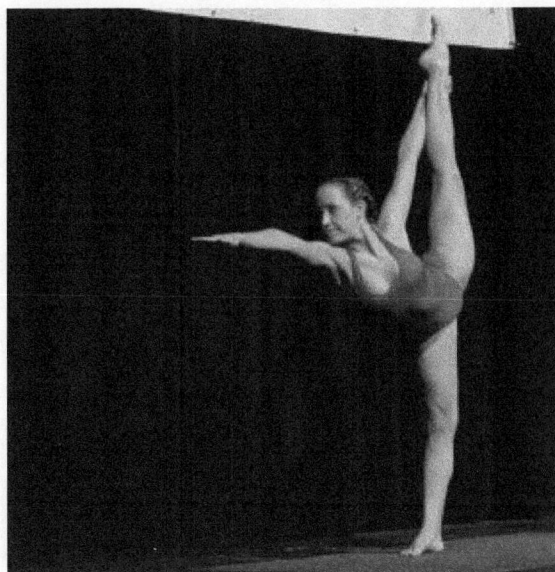

Dancer Split

Be sure you have your balance on your planted foot before getting into a dancer's split.

Reach with your hand to the foot you'll be raising and hold the ankle for balance. Move it slowly behind you and into the air, pausing when needed to regain your balance on your planted side. Once your leg is extended as far as it will go, slowly reach in front of you with the opposite arm.

Keep your upper body curved in this position for added reach.

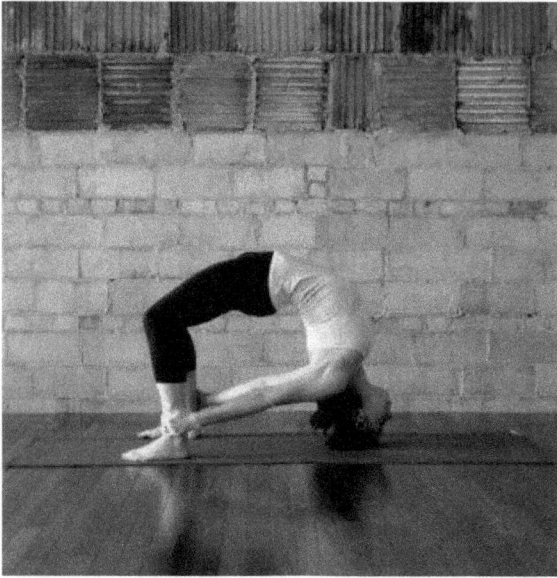

Headstand Bow

Not quite a headstand and not quite a curve, this move is best done from a reclined position.

Curve backwards and reach for your ankles, then push yourself up and outward. Don't hold your body weight with your back but with your leg muscles, resting gently on your head as well.

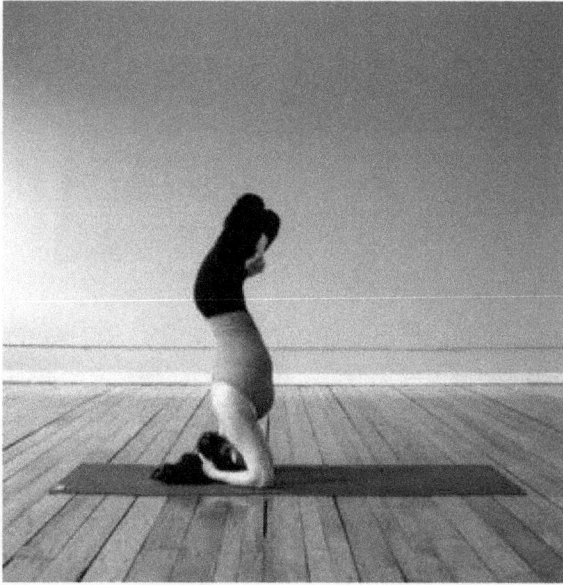

Headstand Lotus

Try this pose against a wall if you're not ready for a headstand. Once you're balanced on your arms and elbows, gently fold one leg down, keeping the other outstretched for balance. Then gently fold down the other leg, taking time to ensure you don't tip in either direction.

Don't use your back to keep yourself in place but push up and back with your arms instead, so you don't pull muscles or strain any area of the back.

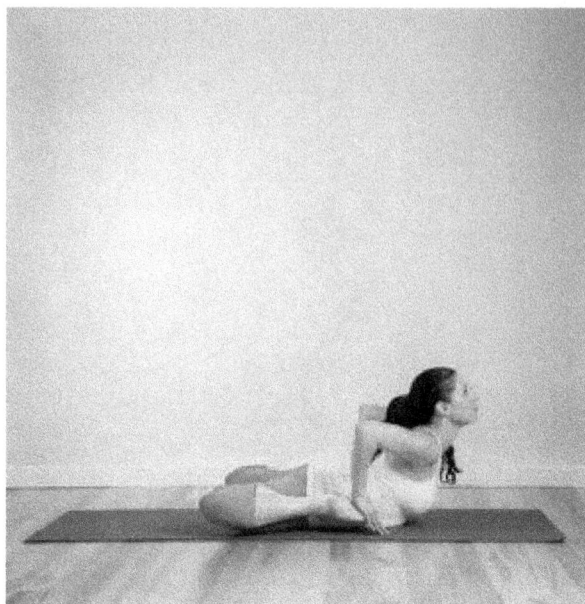

Frog Pose

Pull your feet forward as far as they will go in frog pose, being sure to keep them off the mat and tucked into your body.

If you cannot support yourself with your feet off the mat, allow the legs to stay reclined but active; don't simply collapse your lower body onto the mat. Gently lift and curve your head and neck back and up once you have your balance with your lower body.

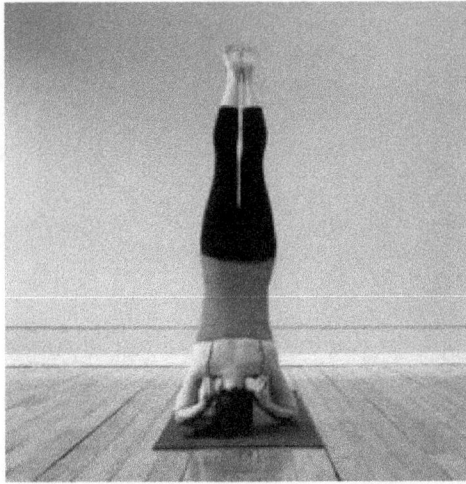

Pinching Shoulders Headstand

This headstand is particularly challenging because your hands are off the mat, so you're holding yourself up with the strength of your lower body and arms alone.

Be sure you're not letting your body push down on your head and neck, and keep your legs upright and balanced before you pick up your hands.

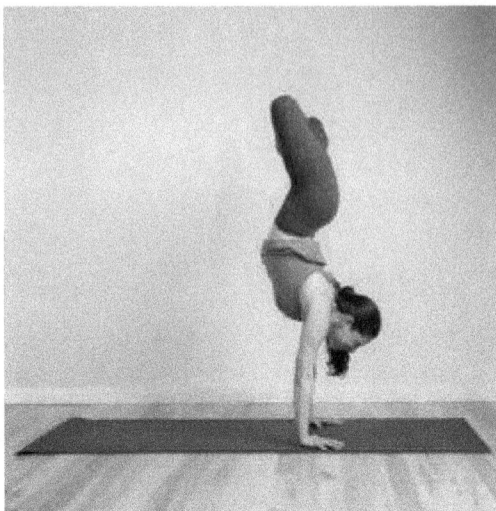

Handstand Lotus

Try this position against a wall or with a friend before doing it on your own, if you're not ready for a full handstand.

While still on your arms and head on the mat, extend your legs and then cross them together. Gently push up with your arms and reach as far as you can with your thigh muscles and hamstrings.

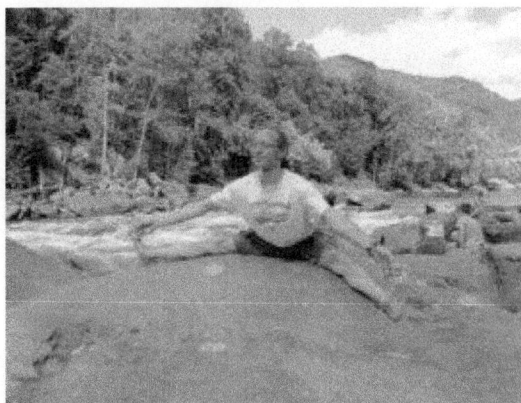

Seated Angle Bend

This is a pose that you should try to make as challenging as possible every time you use it.

Lift your leg with your hand under your knee for support and gently guide it into position, then do the same with the other leg. Bend forward slightly but don't put pressure on the lower back to reach your toes.

If you can't touch your feet, keep your hands in front of you, between your legs, and slide them out as far as possible.

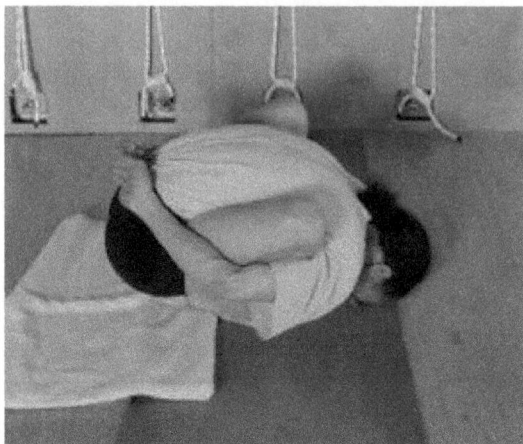

Garland Pose

Start this pose by standing and then bend at the knees and lean forward until your head touches the mat.

For beginners, keep your hands on the mat for balance. When you do get your balance and strength, reach your hands behind you and clasp them together.

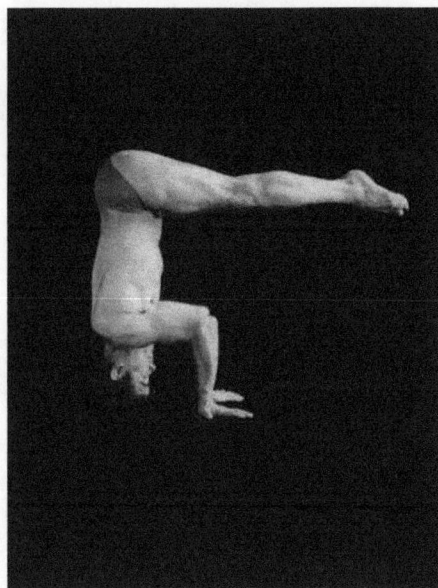

Half Headstand Pose

This pose is very difficult because extending your legs in this position will pull you out of the headstand. Note the turned palms, which help to keep you upright.

Be sure to use the muscles in the thighs and buttocks to pull you toward your back, keeping you in the headstand as you point and extend your legs.

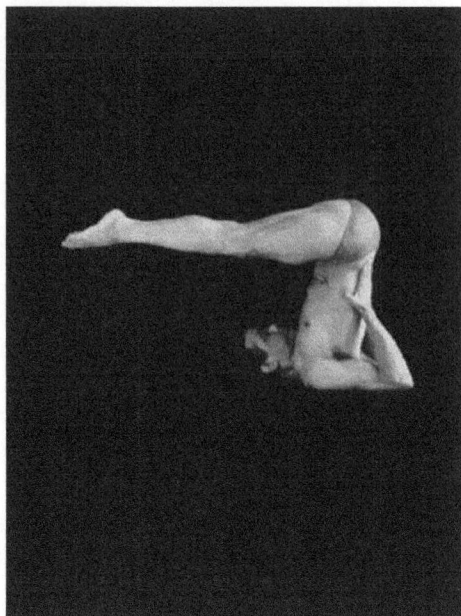

Half Shoulder Stand

This pose can actually be easier than you realize. Use your hands to push your hips up and into place, and use your leg muscles to extend your legs up and over behind you.

It can also be good to use a wall or chair to hold or anchor your feet while you get stronger and better able to hold this position.

Also, be sure to keep your hands in place when you curl out, so you're not putting pressure on your spine.

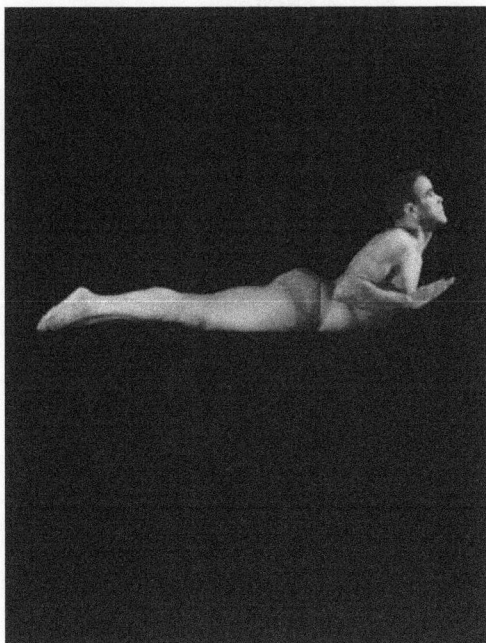

Cobra Pose II

Cobra pose is good for stretching your back and spine, but once you're ready for something advanced try this secondary pose. In the curved position, gently lift your hands off the mat and balance yourself on your legs alone.

This will flex and tense the abdominals as well as stretching the back and leg muscles.

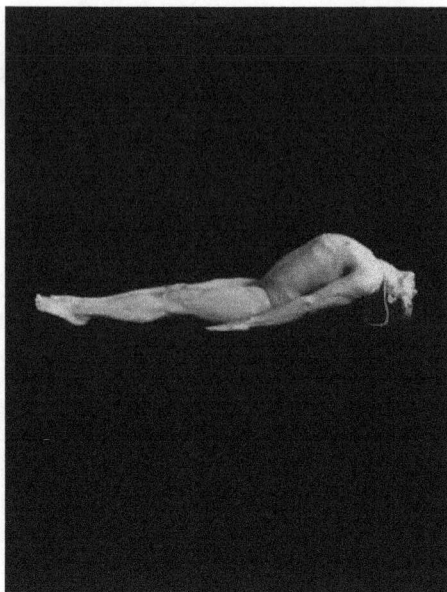

Easy Fish pose

This pose isn't as easy as the name would have you think; drag your head along the mat until the top of your head is touching the ground. Keep your legs straight and active, your palms flat on the mat.

Your abdominals will work to keep you steady while the move will open your chest for better breathing, and stretch your intestines and other parts of your digestive system.

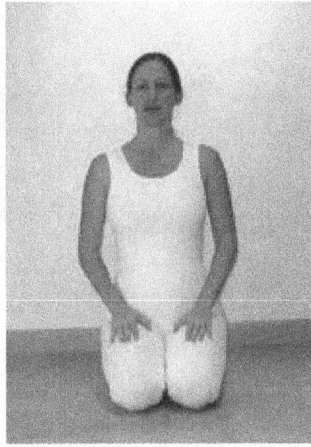

Zen Pose

Zen pose looks very easy but this actually stretches the muscles of the legs. It's a good choice for between movements if you need to recheck your posture and give your body a break from twisting and stretching, and for ending a routine when you want to incorporate a few minutes of meditation into your yoga.

Be sure you keep your back upright in Zen pose and breathe deeply, for maximum benefit.

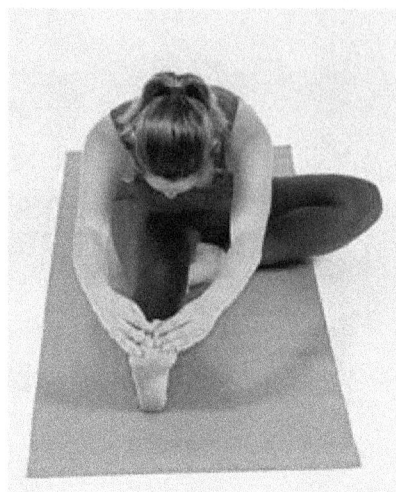

Hand to Knee Pose

Use your hands to guide one leg into position, and remember to tuck your foot onto your thigh and not next to the knee joint.

Gently curve forward rather than just bending; it can help to slide your hands onto the mat for balance as you reach for the foot of the extended leg. Bend onto that leg as deeply as possible for maximum stretching.

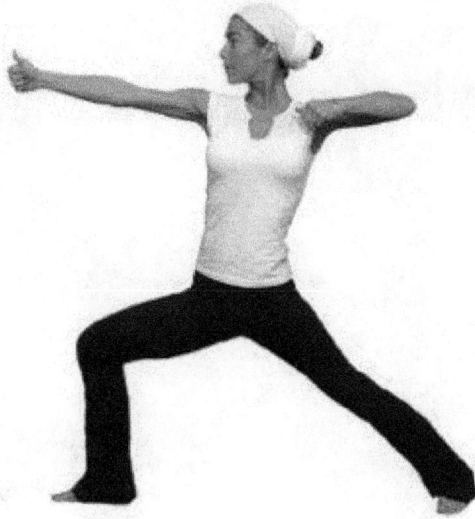

Archer Pose

Step back with one foot and gain your balance, keeping your planted foot straight. Be sure the extended leg is also straight and that you're not bending at the knee. Keep the arms up and pull one behind you, as if pulling a bow.

Mind your posture and breathe deeply to hold this pose.

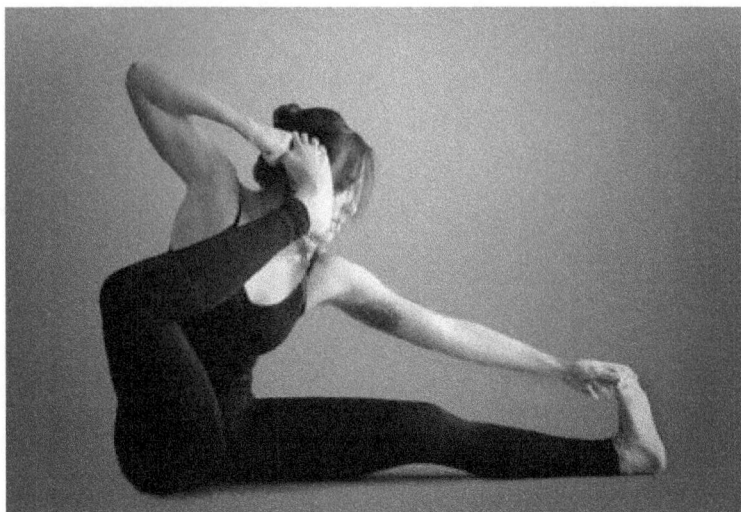

Archer II Pose

Use your hand to guide one leg to the side of your face, keeping that arm bent behind you. Reach forward and touch the toes of the other foot, keeping the back curved.

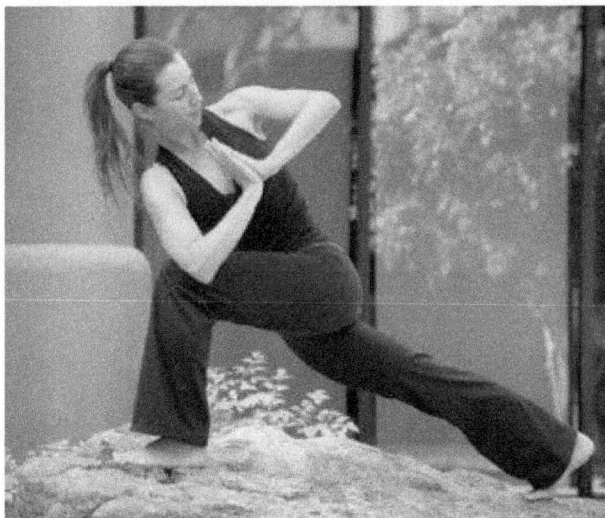

Runner's Lunge with Twist

A lunge works your entire set of leg muscles and helps improve your balance, and a twist makes it even more challenging. Tuck your elbow behind your outer knee to keep you in place, and use both legs to maintain your balance.

Be sure you're leaning into the heel of the planted foot and not your knee.

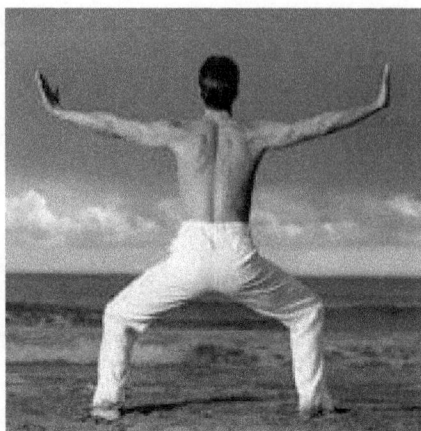

Horse Pose

Horse pose is actually harder than you think, as you need to lean back on your heels to keep pressure off the knees and use all the inner thigh muscles to keep yourself balanced.

Extending the arms also means more of a challenge for being balanced. Keep the buttocks tense and you'll have a firm backside from this pose in no time!

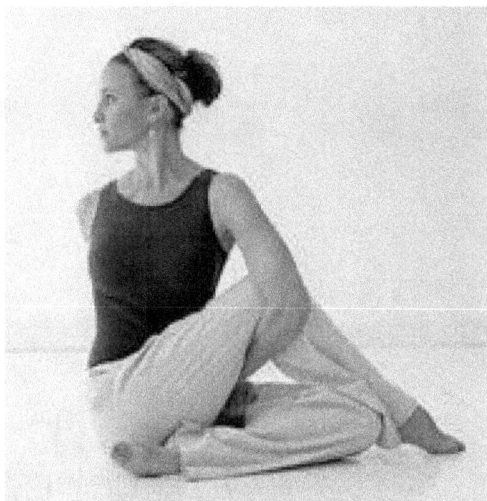

Half Lord of the Fish

Use your hands to pick up one leg and place that foot over the other, crossed leg, then gently twist at the waist and hold both hands together.

Be sure to keep your back upright so you don't put pressure on those muscles, and keep the leg muscles active as well to help keep you in position.

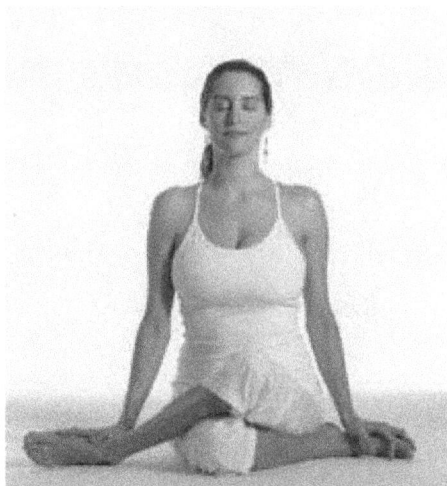

Hero's Pose

Hero's pose stretches the leg muscles and the back, as crossing your knees like this forces you to sit up straight and be aware of your posture.

You can put your hands on the mat next to you in order to keep yourself upright and balanced, or push down on your outside knee very gently for an added stretch.

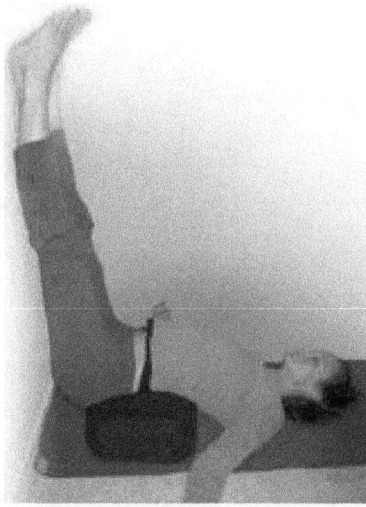

Supported Leg Pose

Putting your legs up against a wall like this stretches your back muscles, but putting a foam block or pillow under the back can give you added support if this position is uncomfortable.

Be sure you relax the back muscles in this pose rather than keeping them tense. The legs should also be extended but relaxed, not tense.

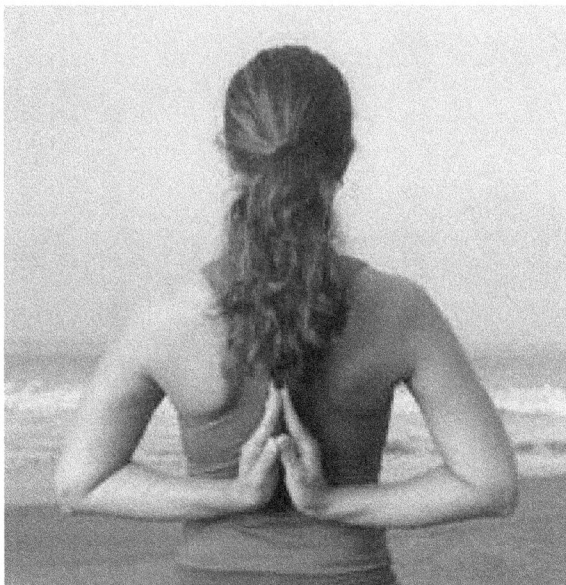

Reverse Namaste

This position looks very simple but it's a great way to open up the chest and clear obstructed breathing passages, and ensure good posture.

Push your hands together for added stretch of the arms and curve the back slightly, pushing out the chest, for a good stretch of those muscles.

Final Words

I would like to thank you for purchasing my book and I hope I have been able to help you and educate you on something new.

If you have enjoyed this book and would like to share your positive thoughts, could you please take 30 seconds of your time to go back and give me a review on my Amazon book page.

I greatly appreciate seeing these reviews because it helps me share my hard work.

You can leave me a review on Amazon.com.

Again, thank you and I wish you all the best!

Enjoying this book?

Check out our other best sellers!

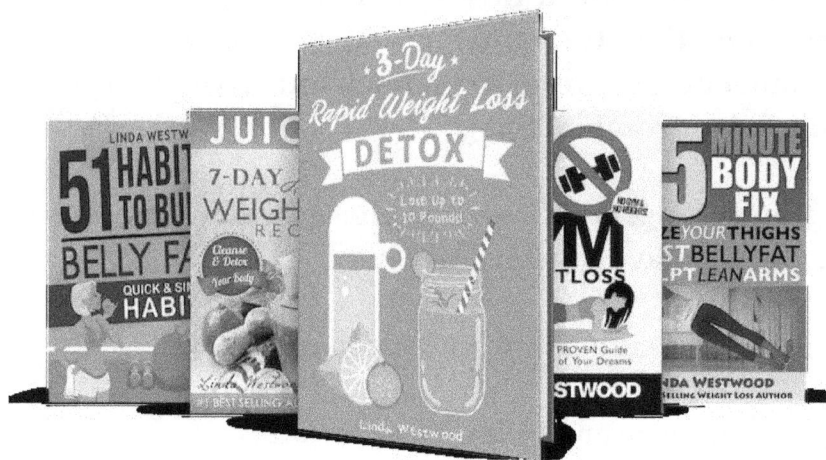

Get your next book on sale here:

TopFitnessAdvice.com/go/books

www.ingramcontent.com/pod-product-compliance
Lightning Source LLC
Chambersburg PA
CBHW031154020426
42333CB00013B/663